The Personalized Nutrition Guide to

Menopause

RESET, RENEW AND REBALANCE THE BODY AND MIND

Christine Bailey

SINGING DRAGON

LONDON AND PHILADELPHIA

by the same author

Eat to Get Younger
Tackling Inflammation and
Other Ageing Processes for
a Longer, Healthier Life
Lorraine Nicolle and Christine Bailey
ISBN 978 1 84819 179 2
eISBN 978 0 85701 125 1

**The Functional
Nutrition Cookbook**
Addressing Biochemical
Imbalances through Diet
Lorraine Nicolle and Christine Bailey
ISBN 978 1 78592 991 5
eISBN 978 0 85701 052 0

of related interest

**Biochemical Imbalances
in Disease**
A Practitioner's Handbook
*Edited by Lorraine Nicolle
and Ann Woodriff Beirne*
ISBN 978 1 84819 033 7
eISBN 978 0 85701 028 5

**Case Studies in
Personalized Nutrition**
Edited by Angela Walker
ISBN 978 1 84819 394 9
eISBN 978 0 85701 351 4

First published in Great Britain in 2026 by Singing
Dragon, an imprint of Jessica Kingsley Publishers
Part of John Murray Press

1

A CIP catalogue record for this title is available from
the British Library and the Library of Congress

ISBN 978 1 80501 144 6
eISBN 978 1 80501 145 3

Printed and bound in China by RR Donnelley

Jessica Kingsley Publishers' policy is to use
papers that are natural, renewable and recyclable
products and made from wood grown in sustainable
forests. The logging and manufacturing processes
are expected to conform to the environmental
regulations of the country of origin.

Singing Dragon
Carmelite House
50 Victoria Embankment
London EC4Y 0DZ

www.singingdragon.com

John Murray Press
Part of Hodder & Stoughton Limited
An Hachette UK Company

The authorised representative in the EEA is
Hachette Ireland, 8 Castlecourt Centre, Dublin
15, D15 XTP3, Ireland (email: info@hbgi.ie)

Contents

Introduction

Menopause is an inevitable transition for all women, but it can also be unpredictable. Whether it's sudden hot flashes, sleepless nights, mood swings and/or the appearance of stubborn belly fat, these changes can leave women feeling out of control. While the range of symptoms can be extensive, what is often overlooked is the power that diet and lifestyle can have in empowering women to feel their most vital self during this time of transition.

Whether you are a health professional guiding your clients through menopause, or an individual seeking to better understand and manage your own symptoms, this comprehensive guide and recipe book, with clear evidence-based strategies and advice, offers practical tools to help you thrive before, during and beyond the menopause.

The aim of this book is to provide dietary and lifestyle recommendations, with easy-to-follow recipes that address both menopausal symptoms and support long-term wellbeing. For practitioners, the book provides a robust framework to support your clients through the menopause transition. With clear explanations of the hormonal changes at play and how they affect different body systems, you'll be equipped with the knowledge to recommend targeted interventions that can significantly improve both immediate symptoms and long-term health outcomes. With the accompanying Reset meal plan and a wealth of recipes (see Part 5 and the Appendix), you will be able to offer practical solutions to enhance your client's energy, support their metabolic health and address their longer-term health concerns.

For women experiencing menopause, this book is your guide to taking control of your health and how to thrive during this natural transition.

Wherever you are in your menopause journey, the insights and strategies will help you manage symptoms more effectively and feel more energized and vibrant. From improving body composition and reducing inflammation to boosting mental clarity and mood, this book offers a comprehensive approach to menopause health.

By combining expert knowledge with practical applications, this book is a valuable resource for anyone seeking to make this stage of life healthier, happier and more fulfilling. So, whether you are a practitioner looking for tools to support your clients or a woman eager to live better through the menopause years, this book is designed for you.

LIVING BETTER THROUGH THE MENOPAUSE YEARS

Menopause is a natural and inevitable transition for women. No matter where you are in your menopause journey, there are dietary and lifestyle changes you can put into action *now* to enable you to thrive during the menopause transition and beyond. Starting with perimenopause, these natural phases in a woman's life involve a complete hormone transformation that can bring with it many health challenges. Not everyone experiencing menopause notices every change or symptom, but by understanding these changes, why they occur and how best to address them, you will be more able to proactively take steps to alleviate symptoms and improve your overall health, vitality and wellbeing. I truly believe there is no reason why your menopausal years shouldn't be the happiest and most fulfilling of your life.

While there is often much attention given to acute symptoms such as hot flashes, brain fog, loss of libido or poor sleep, the menopause transition is fundamentally about the permanent loss of ovarian hormones and the impact this has on the whole body. In fact, the decline in hormones impacts all body systems, and with it major changes occur including inflammation, immune dysregulation and metabolic changes. This, in turn, contributes to an increased risk of various health conditions such as bone and musculoskeletal conditions, heart disease and stroke, type 2 diabetes and alterations in mood and cognitive health.

The good news is that diet, nutrition and lifestyle factors have a profound impact on both long-term health and the more immediate menopause symptoms. During this time of transition, nutrient intake and dietary and lifestyle patterns need to adapt to support this changing health status. It is more important than ever to optimize diet and nutrient intake to support health and vitality in the long term.

While every woman's menopause journey is different, diet, lifestyle and exercise habits can have a dramatic impact on the menopause experience and long-term health outcomes. We are unique, and while there is no one diet that suits everyone, there are some key dietary and lifestyle concepts that can help in addressing the hormone changes that arise during the menopause transition (see the recipes in Part 5 and the meal plans in the Appendix).

Whether you want to improve your body composition, lose fat and enhance muscle mass, feel more energized or have more focus, this book is for you. It is never too late or too early to make positive changes. While the earlier you start, the more likely you are to notice an easier transition, whatever stage you are at, I encourage you to be proactive and take steps to enjoy and thrive during the menopause years and beyond.

HOW TO USE THIS BOOK

This nutrition and recipe guide is more than just a resource – it's also a toolkit for understanding the body, optimizing health and crafting personalized eating plans for this transformative phase of life.

The introductory chapters look at the science behind menopause, the hormonal shifts it brings and how these changes contribute to a wide range of symptoms. We then look at long-term health concerns including metabolic health and weight gain, heart health, cognitive function, emotional wellbeing and bone health, with detailed information and advice enabling you to make informed decisions about wellbeing.

Central to this book is the importance of nutrition and lifestyle, with clear advice and strategies to personalize your approach. After Parts 1 and 2, which look more broadly at what menopause is and optimizing health in the long term, Part 3 includes practical advice and tools around movement and exercise, stress management and optimizing sleep, while Part 4 outlines the underlying principles of how to eat during the menopause transition and beyond. For personalized diet guidance, you will find a Reset stage aimed at improving metabolic health and facilitating weight loss, and a Renew stage for sustained wellness.

In Part 5, you will find recipes to enhance mental clarity and cognition, heart health and bone health. The recipe and meal plan sections are organized to make healthy eating effortless. Recipes are labelled to indicate their benefits for Reset (weight loss and metabolic health), bone health, brain health and heart health or Renew (sustained wellness). They are also marked Vegetarian, Vegan or Gluten free. Use these to design daily meals and snacks around your priorities.

Think of this book as your personal wellness coach, here to help you navigate menopause with confidence. By combining in-depth information, practical tips and delicious recipes, it will equip you to create a sustainable, nourishing plan that supports health and vitality.

Let's make this journey one of empowerment and renewal!

PART 1

WHAT DO WE MEAN BY MENOPAUSE?

Menopause officially starts one year after a woman's final menstrual period. However, while a useful marker, menopause is actually an ongoing and gradual process involving ovarian ageing and accompanied by hormonal decline that impacts all organs and body systems. Menopause is not just the loss of fertility and periods; it signals the beginning of major metabolic and hormonal shifts in a woman's body. It is better to view this phase in life as a hormonal transition rather than an end point. Some symptoms, for example, may be more evident in the first ten years or early menopause, while medical conditions often associated with ageing may occur in later years.

The average age of natural menopause is 51, but it can vary significantly from one woman to another. Some women enter early menopause in their early 40s. For other women who have premature ovarian insufficiency (POI), menopause takes place much earlier, in their 20s or 30s. Other women may enter premature menopause due to surgery (e.g., removal of ovaries and/or uterus) or having undergone cancer treatments such as chemotherapy.

While several hormones undergo shifts during perimenopause and menopause, probably the most profound is that of oestrogen. Nearly every tissue and organ in the body, including the heart, immune system, skin, muscle, brain, bone, breast and digestive tract, has oestrogen receptors, which is why physical and psychological changes occur throughout the body when oestrogen levels fluctuate and then decline dramatically at menopause.

Oestrogen doesn't completely disappear after menopause. It is so crucial for a woman's health that other organs such as the adrenal glands, adipose tissue and brain make oestrogen. However, the main form of oestrogen post menopause is oestrone rather than oestradiol, which is a much weaker form of oestrogen.

PERIMENOPAUSE

Perimenopause is when the body starts the transition to menopause. It begins when ovarian hormone production starts to fall due to a drop in egg stores and the woman no longer ovulates every month. The decline in hormone production impacts the menstrual cycle, often making periods more erratic – they may get shorter in frequency or longer or just unpredictable. As the ovaries release less oestrogen and become less responsive to hormonal signals, the pituitary gland increases the production of follicle-stimulating hormone (FSH) and luteinizing hormone (LH). The appearance of high levels of FSH and LH is characteristic of the perimenopause and often precedes the sustained loss of sex hormone secretion by the ageing ovary.

Perimenopause normally starts in the mid-40s, but can be highly variable. It can last anywhere from two to ten years, although four is more common. As perimenopause progresses, it is common for women to notice a shortening of the menstrual cycle, with a shorter luteal phase and lower progesterone levels. The loss of luteal phase progesterone causes menstrual irregularity, while the subsequent decrease and fluctuations of oestrogen due to follicular exhaustion are associated with other symptoms, including cravings and weight gain. The fluctuations in ovarian hormones can impact the whole body and contribute to the onset of vasomotor symptoms such as hot flashes.[1] Additionally, a relative increase in androgens, such as testosterone, may lead to increased sebum production, contributing to skin changes and acne.

Chapter 1

A Look at the Key Hormones

Hormones are chemical messengers delivering important information to cells throughout your body. They are produced by specific glands, influencing the function and activity of various organs and body systems. They do not work in isolation but exist in a delicate balance, like musical instruments within an orchestra. Throughout the day, various hormones will fluctuate in rhythm with one another. For example, cortisol (a key stress hormone) follows a daily rhythm, rising to its peak in the early morning to help you feel alert and energized, and falling to its lowest levels at night, which supports the rise of melatonin (the hormone that facilitates sleep). The conductor of this orchestra is your brain – in particular, certain areas in the brain such as the hypothalamus and pituitary gland. Your brain communicates to your endocrine organs, including your ovaries, adrenal glands, pancreas and thyroid, to maintain this delicate balance. The trouble is that many factors can affect this balance – stress, your environment, the food choices you make, exercise, sleep patterns and then, of course, the additional hormone shifts that occur around menopause.

Here is a more detailed look at the hormones at play.

OESTROGEN

Oestrogen is much more than a hormone for reproduction; it is a master metabolic hormone that influences immune function, digestion, cardiovascular health, mood and brain function. This makes natural sense since for health and reproduction all these systems need to be functioning optimally. Of course, that also means that when both oestrogen and progesterone decline, you can notice the impact throughout your body. It also explains why certain health conditions such as cardiovascular health risk increase post menopause.[1]

There are three types of oestrogen: oestradiol, oestrone and oestriol. Oestradiol is the main hormone prevalent in women from puberty until menopause. After menopause, oestrone becomes the primary form of oestrogen in the body, produced mainly through the conversion of adrenal androgens, in fat tissue and other peripheral tissues via the enzyme aromatase. Oestriol, the weakest form of oestrogen, is primarily produced during pregnancy.

Oestrogen levels vary throughout the monthly menstrual cycle, being highest at ovulation – around days 12–14 of the cycle – and lowest at menstruation (also known as a 'period') – usually on days 1–5 of the cycle. Oestrogen starts to fall with age and fluctuates after the age of 35 before a sharp decline at menopause. While oestrogen is produced primarily by the ovaries, it is also produced peripherally from cholesterol-derived precursors. Did you know, for example, that oestrogen is so important to the brain that the brain can make its own?

As oestrogen is the master hormone optimizing body functions for reproduction, it plays a key role in metabolic health since this is essential for successful reproduction and survival. Oestrogen can bind to oestrogen receptors throughout the body, influencing their function. In fact, oestrogen plays many roles in various body systems, including supporting musculoskeletal health, digestive function, immune health, cardiovascular health and brain function. Its role in metabolic health[2] explains why, as it declines at menopause, you can experience symptoms such as fatigue, weight gain, belly fat and alterations in your lipid health.[3]

Receptors for oestrogen are found everywhere throughout the body. This is why, as oestrogen levels decline, the effects are evident in a host of body systems and organs. There are a number of different oestrogen receptors, and the two most researched are oestrogen alpha and oestrogen beta. Oestrogen can also activate rapid signals that act within seconds or minutes via extranuclear and membrane-associated forms of oestrogen receptor.[4]

These receptors are distributed differently within your organs. For example, oestrogen alpha is expressed particularly in the reproductive organs – for example, the uterus, ovary, breast – regions in the brain such as the hypothalamus and immune cells including mast cells (involved in immune reactions and releasing compounds such as histamine). Oestrogen beta is expressed throughout the body including the gastrointestinal tract, bone marrow, vascular endothelium, lung, bladder, various immune cells and particularly in many regions of the brain.

One of the reasons why dietary phytoestrogens[5] (see Chapter 11) can be beneficial for women around menopause, particularly in reducing some of the common symptoms like hot flushes, is that they bind to these receptors, having a mild oestrogenic effect.[6]

PROGESTERONE

Progesterone, along with oestrogen, influences menstruation and reproduction. It also helps to maintain a viable pregnancy. Progesterone levels start to decline in the mid-30s and beyond. For many women, the increased fluctuations in oestrogen combined with lower progesterone during the late 30s and into the 40s result in premenstrual syndrome (PMS)-like symptoms such as migraines, irritability and anxiety.

Progesterone interacts with an inhibitory brain neuromodulator known as GABA (gamma-aminobutyric acid). This can have a calming effect on the brain, helping you to feel relaxed and able to unwind. So, as levels of progesterone decline, some women may notice mood changes, sleep disturbances and increased anxiety.

Stress can impact progesterone levels. Although progesterone is mostly made in the ovaries, before menopause a small amount is produced via the adrenal glands where it can be made from pregnanolone (the main precursor from which all sex hormones are derived). However, the adrenal glands can also convert progesterone into the stress hormone cortisol if required. As a result, chronic stress can impact levels of progesterone. This becomes particularly relevant as you transition through menopause, since you will become more reliant on your adrenal glands to support overall levels of progesterone. The more stressed you are, the more those prehormones – pregnanolone and progesterone – can be used to make cortisol. This is why, if you are looking to maintain healthy progesterone levels through perimenopause and menopause, managing stress is critical.

TESTOSTERONE

Testosterone is not just important for men. While oestrogen is the most abundant gonadal hormone during the reproductive years, testosterone is considered the most abundant gonadal androgen in women over the course of their lifespan,[7] and is crucially important for women's health and vitality.

Women make testosterone in their ovaries and in cells within the adrenal glands, fat, skin and brain. In fact, a young women's ovaries produce approximately three to four times more testosterone than oestrogen daily.[8] Around menopause, this means, of course, that symptoms of testosterone deficiency can become noticeable, and the adrenal glands play a bigger role in maintaining levels of this hormone.

Just as for oestrogen, there are receptors for testosterone throughout the body. Testosterone plays a key role in cognition and mood, sex drive, energy, body composition, muscle mass and bone health.[9] This is one of the reasons why, as levels decline, your ability to maintain strength and muscle mass can become more difficult.

The main precursors for testosterone production in the adrenal glands are DHEA (dehydroepiandrosterone) and DHEAS (dehydro-epiandrosterone sulphate). Levels of both testosterone and DHEA begin to decline from the mid- to late 20s. Levels of DHEA can also be influenced by chronic stress. The drop in testosterone precedes menopause with the exception of surgical menopause (when the ovaries are removed), but it is more gradual than the more noticeable drop in oestrogen.

The amount of free testosterone is what is biologically active. This can be influenced by the level of sex hormone binding globulin (SHBG) as this binds up testosterone (and other sex hormones), making less free testosterone available. If you have higher levels of SHBG, there is less available free testosterone – which is not necessarily beneficial around menopause. There are a number of reasons why some people have higher SHBG levels than others. For example, high SHBG is associated with a lower protein diet and blood sugar imbalances (diabetes). This is one of the reasons why dietary changes such as increasing daily protein, including sufficient healthier fats and avoiding sugar and refined carbohydrates can impact testosterone levels.

As testosterone is made from DHEA (in the adrenal glands), paying attention to your stress levels and ensuring sufficient sleep is important to maintain healthy levels. Exercise, particularly resistance training, can also be useful in supporting testosterone levels and, of course, has the additional benefit of supporting muscle mass and bone health. There are also various micronutrients required for the production of testosterone, including zinc, magnesium, vitamins C, K and E, B vitamins and vitamin D. This is why both dietary and lifestyle intervention can impact testosterone levels.

CORTISOL, DHEA, THYROID

Stress can impact progesterone levels in several ways. Although progesterone is primarily made in the ovaries, a small amount is also produced by the adrenal glands. The adrenal glands derive progesterone from pregnenolone, which is the precursor for several steroid hormones.

However, when the body is under stress, the adrenal glands increase cortisol production, the primary stress hormone. This heightened demand for cortisol can reduce the production of other hormones, including progesterone. This occurs because the body uses shared precursors, like pregnenolone, to make both cortisol and sex hormones. As more pregnenolone is directed toward cortisol production, less is available for the synthesis of progesterone.

This becomes particularly relevant during perimenopause and menopause when ovarian hormone production declines, and the body increasingly relies on the adrenal glands for hormone production. Therefore, managing stress becomes critical for maintaining healthy progesterone levels as you navigate perimenopause and menopause.[10]

Prolonged high cortisol can also impact thyroid function – slowing metabolism and contributing to weight gain, fatigue, and cognitive issues – further complicating the hormonal picture during this life stage.

During perimenopause, age, along with declining oestrogen and progesterone, can influence thyroid function by reducing hepatic production of thyroxine-binding globulin (TBG), impairing the peripheral conversion of thyroxine (T4) to triiodothyronine (T3), and potentially increasing thyroid-stimulating hormone (TSH) levels. These changes may contribute to subclinical or overt hypothyroidism and worsen symptoms such as fatigue, mood swings and hot flashes. Fluctuations in sex hormones may also impact immune regulation, potentially unmasking autoimmune thyroid conditions like Hashimoto's thyroiditis in genetically predisposed individuals. Monitoring of thyroid function may be useful to distinguish between menopausal symptoms and underlying thyroid issues.[11]

GROWTH HORMONE

Growth hormone (GH) is often referred to as the 'build-up' hormone because it supports lean muscle mass, bone strength, and helps promote fat breakdown. In adults, GH is involved with muscle repair and recovery and bone mineralization. It can help keep you lean and maintain a healthy body composition. Levels of GH gradually decline as we age. Unfortunately, in women oestrogen regulates GH secretion and modulates the tissue response to GH.[12] This means that after menopause there is a more noticeable decline in GH. The good news is that lifestyle factors can positively impact levels, particularly ensuring sufficient quality sleep and daily exercise (see Chapters 7 and 8). Managing stress (Chapter 9) is equally important, since DHEA can also impact GH levels during menopause.

INSULIN

Insulin signals to tissues such as muscles, the liver and fat cells to absorb glucose from the bloodstream, which can then be used for energy production or stored for later use. In muscles and the liver, glucose is stored as glycogen, while in fat cells, glucose can be converted into fat and stored as triglycerides. Because of its role in promoting energy storage, insulin is often referred to as a 'fat storage hormone'.

However, insulin's effects on overall body fat levels are more complex. While it inhibits fat breakdown (lipolysis) and encourages fat storage, this process is part of a broader hormonal and metabolic system. Several factors influence how insulin affects fat storage, including the macronutrient balance in your diet (protein, fats and carbohydrates), activity levels and overall caloric intake.

One of the problems around menopause, however, is that the decline in oestrogen increases your risk of insulin resistance. This can make your body less responsive to insulin, which can lead to the accumulation of belly (visceral) fat and impaired lipid metabolism. Long term, this can increase your risk of diabetes and cardiovascular disease. In fact, menopausal women are three times more likely to develop obesity and metabolic syndrome than premenopausal women.[13] Studies have also shown that hormone replacement therapy (HRT) in menopausal women can lower visceral adipose tissue, fasting serum glucose and insulin levels. That doesn't mean, of course, that you have to take HRT (see Chapter 12); diet and lifestyle factors can also play a key role in managing blood glucose levels and improving insulin sensitivity. It does, however, emphasize the importance of addressing your metabolic health and in particular improving insulin sensitivity around menopause. This is what the Reset stage of the menopause plan seeks to address (see Part 4).

Chapter 2

Menopause Symptoms and Quality of Life

There is no doubt from the research that menopausal symptoms have a substantial effect on the quality of life of women.[1] Some studies have cited that around 50 per cent of menopausal women are reported to have poor quality of life. It's also estimated that around 86 per cent of women will seek support during the menopausal transition due to the barrage of changes and symptoms arising.[2]

The dramatic impact of hormone changes throughout the body leads to a whole host of symptoms including central nervous system-related disorders; metabolic, weight, cardiovascular, musculoskeletal changes; urogenital and skin atrophy; and sexual dysfunction.[3] Often overlooked are the long-term chronic health risks that increase with menopause, such as diabetes, cardiovascular disease, osteoporosis and Alzheimer's (see Part 2).

For a healthy menopause transition, it is important to address the debilitating symptoms, such as hot flashes, mood changes, joint pain, vaginal dryness and sleep disorders. But you should also be looking to optimize your diet and lifestyle to lower the risk of long-term chronic diseases and enable you to live your life to its fullest during menopause and beyond.

The classic symptoms like hot flushes are typically caused by falling and fluctuating hormone levels, and are often most severe in the perimenopause years. Whether you choose to take hormones (HRT) or not, dietary and lifestyle changes (including optimizing sleep, managing stress and sufficient appropriate exercise) can help your body transition more smoothly.

CENTRAL AND PERIPHERAL NERVOUS SYSTEM

- Cognitive changes (e.g., learning, memory, focus, attention)
- Sleep changes (e.g., insomnia, night sweats, changes to circadian rhythm)
- Mood changes (e.g., more anxiety, irritability, depression)
- Peripheral nerve changes (e.g., unusual skin sensations, pain and touch sensitivity)
- Migraines and headaches
- Vasomotor symptoms (e.g., hot flushes)

DIGESTIVE HEALTH

- Changes in digestion and gastric function (e.g., changes in gastric motility, changes in bowel habits, indigestion, constipation, heartburn)
- New food sensitivities and intolerance
- Changes to the gut microbiome
- Reduction in microbial diversity

MUSCULOSKELETAL SYSTEM

- Loss of muscle mass
- Loss of bone density
- Slower healing of connective tissues; stiffer connective tissues
- More aches and pains in muscles and joints
- Greater incidence of arthritic conditions

METABOLIC HEALTH AND BODY COMPOSITION

- Changes in glucose metabolism and insulin sensitivity
- Changes in fatty acid metabolism
- Changes in hunger and appetite regulation
- Changes in metabolic health, increased fatigue
- Increased visceral and abdominal adiposity
- Changes in fat distribution
- Greater risk of weight gain
- Increased risk of fatty liver

RESPIRATORY SYSTEM

- Higher risk of respiratory infections and COPD
- Lower lung capacity and function
- Greater risk of allergic reactions

CARDIOVASCULAR SYSTEM

- Stiffer and less elastic blood vessels
- Higher blood pressure
- Higher cardiovascular disease risk
- Increased risk of blood clotting
- Changes in lipid health

IMMUNE FUNCTION

- Higher inflammation and elevated immune response to pro-inflammatory cytokines
- Decreased activity of some immune cell types (e.g., natural killer cells)
- Increased risk of allergies
- Increased risk of autoimmune conditions

SKIN AND HAIR CHANGES

- Thinner, drier skin
- Reduced skin thickness
- Reduced hydration
- Increased wrinkling
- Odd or unusual skin sensations (e.g., formication)
- Acne and outbreaks
- Reduced wound healing
- Thinning hair
- Drier hair
- Hair loss

GENITOURINARY SYMPTOMS

- Vaginal changes (e.g., dryness and thinning skin, lower elasticity, more pain)
- Urogenital changes (e.g., pain when urinating, urinary tract changes)
- Increased risk of pelvic floor dysfunction (e.g., leaking urine)
- Possible sexual dysfunction (e.g., dyspareunia, decreased libido)

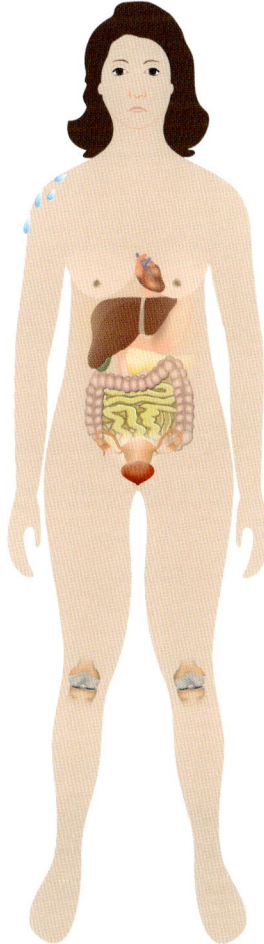

FIGURE 1. BODY SYSTEM CHANGES AT MENOPAUSE[4]

SKIN AND HAIR CHANGES

Acne

While commonly associated with the teenage years, about a quarter of perimenopausal women will develop acne. During the perimenopause, there is a relative increase in androgen hormones, particularly testosterone. This relative increase stimulates the skin to produce more sebum and can make pores seem larger.[5] Other factors such as insulin resistance and thyroid changes can also play a role in acne.

Taking action: The good news is that as you transition from perimenopause to menopause, outbreaks are likely to decline. Reducing refined carbohydrates and increasing your intake of essential fats, plant-based foods, fibre and probiotic-rich foods – which are all key features of the diet plan – can help to improve your skin's appearance.

Wrinkles and dryness

As women approach menopause, skin ageing accelerates.[6] Studies show that women's skin loses about 30 per cent of its collagen during the first five years of menopause. The reduction in oestrogen leads not just to collagen loss but also skin atrophy, reduced skin hydration, decreased skin elasticity and increased wrinkle formation. As collagen and elastin diminishes, the skin loses its firmness and elasticity and begins to sag. Levels of hyaluronic acid, which moisturize the skin and keep it looking plump and glowing, decline. There is also a decline in blood flow to the skin. All these changes result in more noticeable wrinkles, pigmentation and liver spots, and drier and more fragile-looking skin. Many women also notice that bruising is more obvious, and any cuts take longer to heal.

Taking action: Skin needs a balance of essential nutrients for optimal health. It is important to ensure sufficient protein in the diet as well as vitamin C (to support collagen production),[7] antioxidants to protect the skin from damage, essential fats to reduce dryness and foods rich in nitrates to support blood flow. Collagen supplementation may be helpful.[8] Some studies suggest that increasing phytoestrogens such as isoflavones (found in soy products) may be beneficial.[9] Many of the recipes in this book contain foods rich in phytoestrogens.

Hair thinning

It is common in early menopause for women to notice both hair loss and thinning.[10] Hair may also appear finer and break more readily. Vascular changes reducing blood flow to the scalp as oestrogen declines can play a role, and a relative increase in testosterone levels can lead to hair follicle changes and hair loss.[11] Almost 20–60 per cent of women will have noticed significant hair loss before the age of 60.

Taking action: Protein, particularly the sulphur amino acids (cysteine and methionine), is the precursor to keratin hair protein synthesis, so ensure your diet includes quality protein-rich foods. Ensuring sufficient fat, which is required for hormone production (from cholesterol), can also ensure sufficient sebum in the scalp to hydrate the hair. At the same time, keeping refined carbohydrates low has been shown to reduce inflammation and avoid excessive insulin, which may impact blood flow to the scalp. A number of nutrients such as vitamins A, C, D, B vitamins and minerals including iron, zinc, copper and selenium have been shown to influence hair growth and appearance.[12] Scalp massage, red light therapy and platelet-rich plasma therapy are additional therapies that may have some benefit.

DIGESTIVE ISSUES

During menopause, the gut undergoes significant changes due to declining levels of oestrogen and progesterone. These hormones, which have receptors throughout the digestive system, help maintain gut health by regulating processes such as motility, digestion and microbial balance. As oestrogen levels drop, women often experience an increase in digestive issues, including bloating, constipation and irritable bowel syndrome (IBS) symptoms.

One of the major changes is a reduction in gut microbiome diversity, with a decrease in beneficial bacteria such as *Lactobacillus*, *Bifidobacterium* and *Akkermansia*, which are crucial for maintaining gut health, immune function and metabolism.[13] Such changes in the gut microbiota can promote inflammation and increase the risk of gut permeability, where microbes and toxins can pass through the gut lining into the bloodstream, triggering systemic inflammation.[14]

Additionally, hormonal changes impact gut–brain communication, known as the gut–brain axis, exacerbating stress responses and mood swings, which are common during menopause. The decline in oestrogen also affects the production of short-chain fatty acids (SCFAs), such as butyrate, which play a key role in reducing inflammation, supporting gut barrier integrity and regulating metabolism.

Reflux can be more problematic. There is a decline with age in the production of stomach acid, which may impact how well food is broken down.[15] This may have a knock-on effect on the amount of nutrients that can be absorbed in the gut as well as potentially increasing adverse reactions to foods or intolerances. A reduction in stomach acid can be particularly problematic for absorption of iron, which is essential for energy metabolism, and vitamin B12, which supports the nervous system and helps reduce tiredness and fatigue.

Declining oestrogen can also impact motility of the gut, meaning slower transit, while pelvic floor dysfunction can result in incomplete bowel evacuation. The enteric (gut) nervous system, which controls digestion, is sensitive to oestrogen, so as levels decline, you can be more prone to bowel changes, IBS and heartburn.

Taking action: Stress can have a profound effect on the gut microbiome, production of digestive enzymes and stomach acid and motility. Read Chapter 9 on managing stress and take action. Regular exercise can improve motility of the gut, while ensuring sufficient fibre, prebiotics and probiotics in the diet can support a healthier gut microbiome in the longer term. In addition, studies suggest that probiotic supplements[16] may also ease certain menopause symptoms. Our menopause plan has a strong focus on plant-heavy dishes, prebiotics and fermented foods to support gut health.

VASOMOTOR SYMPTOMS

Heart palpitations

Around 25 per cent of menopausal women experience heart palpitations. This is where you may notice your heartbeat increases or its rhythm changes. The heartbeat is controlled by the autonomic nervous system, which, in turn, is influenced by oestrogen. The sympathetic nervous system (involved in the stress response) may be more easily triggered during menopause, which can further exacerbate these symptoms. Such symptoms can occur at any time of the day and may be accompanied by chest pain or sweating. If you experience these symptoms, it is important to get these checked for other underlying conditions.

Taking action: Put in place lifestyle measures such as box breathing, non-sleep deep rest or meditation to switch on the parasympathetic nervous system associated with rest and relaxation (see Chapter 9 on stress). Avoid alcohol and caffeine, which may worsen these palpitations. Exercise regularly and pay attention to blood sugar levels. Certain minerals such as magnesium and potassium may be beneficial.

Hot flashes and night sweats

Hot flashes affect up to 80 per cent of perimenopausal women. They can vary from mild increases in heat to severe flashes accompanied by sweating and palpitations.[17] For most women, hot flashes last for two to three years, but some may experience them for ten years or more.[18] Body temperature regulation is influenced by ovarian hormones, which, in turn, are controlled by the autonomic nervous system. Hot flashes can therefore indicate that the autonomic nervous system has become dysregulated, which may make you more prone to cardiovascular issues, higher blood pressure and palpitations.

Taking action: Surprisingly, exercise can reduce the risk of hot flashes, although you may find certain types of exercise better than others. Spicy foods, alcohol, smoking, caffeine, stress and being overweight may worsen symptoms. Increasing your intake of phytoestrogenic foods (see

Chapter 11) may be beneficial, and consider incorporating box or slow breathing to reduce the stress response. Some studies suggest that a diet high in fruits, vegetables, wholegrains, pulses and legumes, as well as including more fats from oily fish, nuts and seeds, helps manage symptoms.[19] Equally, other studies suggest a more plant-based diet[20] can bring relief from symptoms, particularly one including soybeans, which are a source of phytoestrogens. The isoflavone content of soy foods may be effective in reducing menopausal symptoms. One study recommended 20 mg/day of soy isoflavones supplementation during perimenopause for symptom reduction. This corresponds to 400 ml/day of soy drinks or 80 g/day of other soy products (tofu, tempeh or fermented soy products).[21]

Ginger, while commonly used for easing nausea, can also provide menopause relief. In one study ginger supplementation significantly reduced the intensity of menopausal symptoms, particularly physical symptoms such as hot flashes, night sweats and musculoskeletal pain.[22] Acupuncture may also be beneficial for hot flushes.[23]

MUSCULOSKELETAL SYMPTOMS

Joint pain/arthritis

Arthralgia (joint pain) is experienced by more than half the women around the time of menopause. Oestrogen has anti-inflammatory and protective effects on joint tissues such as cartilage, and various interactions occur between sex hormones and pain-processing pathways as well as immune cells and chondrocytes (cartilage-building cells) to influence joint health.[24] The menopause transition also coincides with rising incidence of chronic rheumatic conditions such as osteoarthritis/rheumatoid arthritis. Oestrogen helps protect articular cartilage from damage, so as levels decline, women may notice old joint injuries flare up or they are more prone to new injuries. During menopause, there is a decline in the production of collagen, elastin and hyaluronic acid, which help to protect cartilage and bones and provide joint lubrication. If you exercise, you may also notice it takes longer for your body to recover after a hard training session; this is because your sex hormones are involved in protein synthesis and muscle repair.

Taking action: Ensure sufficient protein to support bone and joint health. Adding a collagen supplement with vitamin C may be beneficial. Increase your intake of anti-inflammatory omega-3 fats; antioxidants from colourful fruits, vegetables, nuts and seeds as well as isoflavone-rich foods (see Chapter 11) can also be beneficial. Certain supplements such as glucosamine, chondroitin, boswellia, curcumin and omega-3 fatty acids[25] may be beneficial for certain joint conditions.

GENITOURINARY SYMPTOMS

Genitourinary syndrome of the menopause (GSM) refers to a chronic, progressive vulvovaginal, sexual and lower urinary tract condition, which is characterized by several symptoms that may or may not coexist.[26,27] It is estimated to affect 15 per cent of premenopausal women, with up to 65 per cent of women suffering one year after menopause and 84 per cent experiencing symptoms six years after the menopause. Symptoms include vaginal dryness, loss of lubrication, vaginal bleeding and discharge, vulval burning and urinary symptoms such as recurrent urinary tract infections, urge or stress incontinence.[28] The symptoms are due to a reduction in circulating oestrogen, which also impacts the genitourinary microbiome.[29]

Vaginal dryness

The vagina contains oestrogen receptors that regulate lubrication, so when oestrogen levels decline, the walls of the vagina thin and the blood flow declines, resulting in dryness and vagina atrophy.[30] This can contribute to pain during sexual intercourse and leave the vaginal area more prone to irritation and soreness. It can also increase susceptibility to infections.

Taking action: Localized vaginal oestrogen creams are often prescribed, which can also be used with other lubricants. Regular sexual intercourse can improve blood flow to the vagina and improve the muscular tone. Dehydration may exacerbate dryness. Suppositories of vitamins E and D and hyaluronic acid can be beneficial. Sea buckthorn oil,[31] which is rich in essential fatty acids like linolic acid, can strengthen the barrier of the skin and reduce dryness. Ensuring the diet is rich in essential omega-3 and omega-6 fatty acids may also be beneficial.[32]

Bladder issues

Urinary incontinence rates are noticeably higher around menopause. This is usually caused by sphincter or bladder dysfunction, with the most common being stress incontinence, where leakage is caused by a weakened urinary sphincter. An overactive bladder is usually caused by some kind of irritation to the bladder, and results in symptoms of urgency and/or frequency. As oestrogen levels decline, this influences the connective tissue that supports the bladder and urethra. This can result in vaginal prolapse, which weakens the muscles of the urinary tract. In addition, bladder contractions are controlled by the autonomic nervous system, which is also influenced by levels of oestrogen and become dysregulated.

Taking action: In addition to wearing pads, Kegel exercises, nerve stimulation therapy devices and medications can help. Interestingly, studies have also found that vitamin D deficiency is associated with a higher risk of pelvic floor disorders. One study of older women found the risk of developing urinary incontinence was 45 per cent lower among those with normal vitamin D levels. Magnesium may be helpful for supporting muscle and nerve action. Some women find that caffeine[33] and alcohol can irritate the bladder. Cranberry, which is available as a juice or supplement, is rich in proanthocyanidins, and these antioxidants may help prevent urinary tract infections (UTIs), which become increasingly common after menopause.

POOR SLEEP/INSOMNIA

Many women notice a change in their sleep patterns around perimenopause and menopause. This may include difficulty getting to sleep, waking frequently during the night or just not feeling refreshed on waking in the morning. Both oestrogen and progesterone levels can impact sleep. Progesterone, for example, is an anti-anxiety and relaxing hormone, so as levels decline, women may feel more stressed and anxious, and can struggle to wind down at night. Low oestrogen can alter the sleep–wake circadian rhythm, which may mean you wake up too early or struggle to get to sleep. Oestrogen helps the body get into that deep, slow-wave of restorative sleep and influences levels of serotonin (a chemical that is converted to melatonin, which helps you sleep). Less melatonin can result in lighter, more disturbed, sleep patterns. Of course, other symptoms such as hot flashes and heart palpitations can also impact sleep patterns.

Taking action: For practical tips and dietary and lifestyle advice, see Chapter 8 on sleep and the circadian rhythm.

OTHER SYMPTOMS

Due to the presence of oestrogen receptors in all organs and body systems it is no surprise to learn that many other symptoms can manifest during the menopause transition. These include bleeding gums, changes in body odour and breast tenderness as well as dry eyes and macular changes.

PART 2

OPTIMIZING HEALTH LONG TERM

As oestrogen receptors are present throughout the body, playing vital roles in various physiologic functions, the decline of oestrogen around menopause can have longer-term implications for women's health. While we may think of many of these health problems as just signs of ageing, they often begin to show up in conjunction with menopause. By identifying them and taking action, the risk of debilitating health conditions can be reduced, enabling women to feel vibrant and healthy during menopause and beyond.

Common longer-term health concerns include:

- weight gain, obesity and belly fat
- metabolic syndrome, insulin resistance and type 2 diabetes
- musculoskeletal changes – osteoporosis, osteoarthritis
- cardiovascular health and atherosclerosis
- cognitive decline, Alzheimer's disease
- autoimmune diseases (rheumatoid arthritis)
- fatty liver disease
- gastrointestinal disorders – reflux, IBS, constipation
- mood disorders – depression and anxiety
- insomnia.

Perimenopause and menopause is an inflammatory transition. Oestrogens are a key influence on immune and inflammatory processes. With the decline around menopause, women are more prone to experience increased inflammatory responses to infection, with a higher rate of auto-immune diseases in postmenopausal women when compared to men.[1] It is well known that the decline in the ovarian steroidal hormones (oestrogen and progesterone) enhances the inflammatory process, predisposing menopausal women to immune disorders such as rheumatoid arthritis.[2] This is also seen in increased levels of inflammatory cytokines (chemicals) such as interleukin 6 (IL-6)[3] and tumor necrosis factor (TNF)-alpha.

What does this all mean? The transition through perimenopause and menopause is an inflammatory one, and the associated rise in chronic low-grade inflammation affects the whole body (e.g., heart, metabolic health, brain, bone, joints). One of the benefits of HRT when started early (during perimenopause or the first few years of menopause) is to prevent a dramatic shift in the immune response and inflammatory processes.[4] This also reinforces the importance of starting early when it comes dietary and lifestyle changes to support yourself through this transition and, in particular, taking steps to lower inflammation and support specific body systems.

Laboratory testing can be particularly helpful in identifying any specific health concerns or body systems requiring attention, inflammatory markers and micronutrient status. You may wish to pay specific attention to the heart because heart disease is still the number-one killer of post-menopausal women. The good news is that through dietary and lifestyle intervention, and for some women hormone therapy, you can work to support the whole body and all body systems to improve health and resilience in the long term.

Chapter 3

Tackling Weight Gain and Belly Fat

One of the most common complaints around menopause is not only weight gain but also a gradual accumulation of fat, particularly around the tummy. Despite your best efforts, it feels harder to shift the weight. This change in body composition and shape is in part due to the decline in oestrogen. Oestrogen has numerous actions in different body systems that affect your ability to control your appetite and food intake, blood glucose balance, influence insulin sensitivity and even where your fat is distributed. Addressing these metabolic changes is crucial for long-term health, improving body composition and losing weight.

THE PROBLEM WITH INSULIN RESISTANCE

Oestrogen is a key player when it comes to insulin sensitivity in the female body. As oestrogen levels decline during the menopause transition, the body's ability to respond effectively to insulin can diminish. This contributes to insulin resistance, a condition where cells become less responsive to insulin. This is because oestrogen influences certain cells in the pancreas known as pancreatic islet beta cells, which regulate insulin secretion. When oestrogen levels drop, insulin secretion and regulation can become less efficient. It helps regulate GLUT4 (glucose transporter type 4), which facilitates the uptake of glucose into muscle and fat cells. It influences hepatic glucose production (how much sugar the liver releases into the blood). It modulates lipolysis, the process of breaking down stored fat for energy. As a result, women may have a harder time shuttling blood sugar into their muscles for energy when they need it, and instead have a tendency to increase fat storage, especially in the mid-section.

Research indicates the following changes can occur which impact carbohydrate metabolism during menopause:

- Due to oestrogen decline, the insulin secretion of the pancreatic beta cells decreases.
- Decreased insulin sensitivity in the muscles results in a decrease in glucose uptake.
- As a result of deteriorating insulin sensitivity in the liver, gluconeogenesis (process of producing glucose from non carbohydrates sources like amino acids and fats) and lipogenesis (process by which the body converts extra sugars, especially from carbohydrates, into fat which happens in the liver and fat tissues) increase, triglyceride accumulation increases, VLDL production increases, and insulin clearance decreases.
- As a result of the reduced insulin effect on adipose tissue, lipolysis increases, the size of fat cells increases, and inflammatory mediators accumulate.
- The resulting metabolic changes can increase the risk of developing of metabolic syndrome. (Metabolic syndrome is a cluster of health conditions – including high blood pressure, high blood sugar, excess belly fat and abnormal cholesterol levels that can increase the risk of heart disease and diabetes).[1]

APPETITE

Another action of oestrogen is its influence on hunger and satiety hormones. By acting in an area of the brain called the hypothalamus, oestrogen helps regulate appetite.[2] The hormone leptin, for example, has the ability to shut down appetite, making you feel full. At the same time, the hormone ghrelin increases your sense of hunger and may reduce your fat-burning efficiency and energy expenditure. The decline in both oestrogen and progesterone impacts these two hormones. Levels of your hunger-stimulating hormones go up while levels of your appetite-suppressing hormones go down, leaving you always feeling hungry. To make matters worse, you may find yourself craving high-calorie and higher-fat foods too. Clinical studies have shown that cravings for high-fat, palatable foods, as well as binge-eating episodes, increase in the luteal phase of the menstrual cycle when oestrogen levels are low.[3] So persistently low levels around menopause may make it harder to resist higher-calorie, high-fat foods.

Other factors can play a role. For example, a decline in sleep quantity and quality can influence appetite. Even one night of poor sleep can have negative effects on the body, impacting hunger hormones, glucose balance, energy levels and growth hormone – all of which can affect body composition.[4] Too much stress and the release of hormones like cortisol can also impact appetite and cravings. Even if your overall weight does not change, your body composition may (i.e., you are gaining body fat and losing lean muscle tissue), and this is important for your health.

METABOLISM

To make matters worse, oestrogen impacts the metabolism via its regulation of mitochondrial function (which is involved in energy production).[5] As oestrogen levels decline, mitochondrial function can be impaired. So it should come as no surprise that women find it harder to lose weight around menopause, and feel tired and flabby.

During the period of perimenopause and menopause, due to the change in hormone levels the basal metabolism of the female body decreases significantly, which can mean a decrease in the basal metabolic rate (BMR) of up to 250–300 kcal per day. Without any changes to your diet or lifestyle, this may result in an annual weight gain of 2 kg.[6]

Additionally, oestrogen also plays a role in thyroid hormone metabolism, and as levels drop, this can lead to an increase in thyroid-stimulating hormone (TSH), which may contribute to hypothyroidism. Suboptimal thyroid function further slows metabolism, making it even more difficult for women to maintain or lose weight during menopause, while also exacerbating feelings of fatigue and sluggishness.[7]

Declining oestrogen levels, which contribute to excess belly fat during perimenopause and menopause, compound the effects of muscle tissue loss. This can, in turn, impact the metabolism. The decline in other hormones such as DHEA and testosterone further contributes to body composition changes, resulting in a decline in muscle mass, power and strength. A reduction in muscle mass affects metabolic rate and ability to respond to insulin and manage blood glucose health. Additionally, a menopause-related increase in inflammation marker levels and a decrease in muscle mass have an additive negative impact on metabolic health.[8] Maintaining or even improving muscle mass as we age is vitally important for metabolic health and longevity,[9] which is why having a daily and consistent exercise programme is so important (see Chapter 7).

One of best things you can do for your health is maintain a healthy weight and increase muscle mass.[10] If you are noticing an increase in tummy fat, it's time to take action. Excess body fat increases your risk of various health problems in the long term, including type 2 diabetes, metabolic syndrome, non-alcoholic fatty liver disease and cardiovascular disease. In addition, being overweight can exacerbate other health concerns such as joint issues, and impact your mood and self-confidence. However, the focus should be on optimizing health (physically and mentally) rather than simply the goal of losing weight. This requires a rethink, not only of what and when you eat, but how you can incorporate daily exercise and healthy habits in the long term.

Taking action: If you are looking to change your body composition and lose fat, then starting with the Reset meal plan will be helpful (see the Reset meal plan in the Appendix). During these weeks, you will focus on dietary choices to improve blood sugar and insulin sensitivity. This means minimizing foods with a high glycaemic index such as simple carbohydrates (white flour, pasta, breads, baked goods) and sugars, and focusing more on lean proteins, fibrous, non-starchy vegetables and healthy fats. The aim is to reduce dramatic responses in blood sugar that can lead to an exaggerated insulin response. By including more plant-based foods in the diet, you will boost your intake of fibre, which can increase satiety and support a more diverse gut microbiome. Similarly, sufficient lean protein[11] in the diet will improve feelings of fullness. Variations in the gut microbiome[12] also appear to influence blood glucose responses to food eaten. For example, studies have shown that the bacteria *Akkermansia muciniphila*[13] plays a role in supporting gut barrier function and regulating body weight in both rodents and humans. Increased levels of Akkermansia in people with metabolic disorders have been associated with improved glucose control and insulin sensitivity. Other beneficial microbes, such as Faecalibacterium prausnitzii, produce short-chain fatty acids like butyrate, which help reduce inflammation and improve insulin sensitivity. The gut microbiome also plays a role in stimulating the release of GLP-1 (glucagon-like peptide-1), a hormone that enhances insulin secretion and supports appetite regulation. This is why many of the recipes in this book include fermented foods and prebiotic-rich ingredients (see Part 5).

If you are looking to reduce overall body fat, it can be helpful to limit snacks and avoid drinking your calories with fruit juices, fizzy drinks, café drinks and alcohol. Protein is a critically important macronutrient for supporting muscle mass as well as being effective in reducing cravings, keeping you feeling full for longer and improving metabolic health. Some research suggests that ensuring sufficient protein at breakfast helps reduce cravings later in the day and keeps you feeling full for longer, meaning you are less likely to overeat later. While calories do matter when it comes to weight loss, the recipes in this book also emphasize the quality of the foods you eat (favouring whole, unprocessed foods) and the types of macronutrients (protein, fibre-rich carbs and healthy fats).

When it comes to managing your weight and blood glucose response, remember the importance of lifestyle factors (see Part 3) including stress, exercise and sleep. Stress itself can potentially influence lifestyle choices, including diet and exercise habits, which may contribute to blood glucose changes and weight gain. Exercise, including after meals, is particularly important in this respect (see the exercises in Chapter 7). Research suggests that even short bouts of activity, such as walking for 10–30 minutes after a meal, can significantly improve insulin sensitivity compared to remaining sedentary.[14] Stress also leads directly to glucose dysregulation and increased inflammation in response to chronically elevated cortisol levels – taking steps to manage your stress is therefore important (see Chapter 9 on stress).

CAN SUPPLEMENTS HELP?

Various nutrients[15] are known to improve blood sugar response and insulin sensitivity.[16] These include certain plant compounds[17] including bioflavonoids such as resveratrol (naturally found in berries and cacao powder) and quercetin (e.g., red apples, capers and red cabbage). More specifically, supplements such as alpha lipoic acid,[18,19] berberine and chromium may be beneficial.

While food and lifestyle is always the foundation for metabolic health, certain supplements can serve as valuable tools to help move women towards better metabolic resilience – especially during times of hormonal transition.

An emerging area of interest in metabolic health, particularly relevant during menopause, involves supporting GLP-1 (glucagon-like peptide-1), a hormone released from the gut that enhances insulin secretion, slows gastric emptying and promotes satiety. Certain foods can naturally stimulate GLP-1 release, including protein-rich foods (such as eggs, dairy and fish), resistant starches and fermentable fibres (like oats, legumes, onions and cooked-and-cooled potatoes), and polyphenol-rich foods like berries, green tea and dark chocolate. These fibres also promote the production of butyrate, a short-chain fatty acid produced by gut bacteria, which has been shown to enhance GLP-1 secretion and improve insulin sensitivity. Supplements such as berberine, resveratrol and probiotics may further support this pathway by either stimulating GLP-1 directly or improving the gut environment that regulates its release. Together, these dietary strategies may help mitigate the insulin resistance and weight gain often seen with declining oestrogen levels.

Lipoic acid[20,21] is an antioxidant that has been shown to improve insulin sensitivity, reduce insulin resistance and improve blood sugar control. Berberine[22] is an alkaloid that is extracted from certain botanical herbs, including barberry, goldenseal and Oregon grape. Berberine's mechanism for lowering blood glucose rests in its ability to increase insulin receptor expression.[23] Research suggests that berberine helps stimulate glucose uptake in the muscles.[24] Multiple clinical studies have shown berberine supplementation can lead to a reduction in both blood glucose and improvements in lipid profiles. Note that as berberine has the ability to alter the gut microbiome, it is recommended to seek support from a healthcare practitioner, as it may not be appropriate for everyone or for long-term use.

Chromium[25] is a trace mineral that is often overlooked but of utmost importance for proper blood sugar regulation.[26] Low chromium levels are associated with impaired glucose and insulin function, which can, in turn, lead to type 2 diabetes. Chromium[27] increases insulin receptor numbers and affinity, allowing for increased insulin binding to cells. Chromium[28] also activates intracellular signalling pathways involved in GLUT4 translocation, increasing glucose transport and enhancing insulin sensitivity. Remember that as oestrogen levels decline, it is this transporter system that can be compromised, so chromium supplementation may be beneficial. Foods rich in chromium include grape juice, beef, tomato juice, apples, Brewer's yeast, green beans and orange juice.

Biotin can be an important adjunct vitamin to chromium when it comes to blood sugar regulation. It has been shown to increase the efficacy of chromium when used to address blood glucose levels. In clinical trials, pairing biotin with chromium[29] improved hacmoglobin A1c (HbA1c) and fasting glucose levels, and has led to decreases in current prescription medications for diabetic patients. Combining biotin and chromium may therefore be beneficial when it comes to improving blood sugar balance.

If you are considering taking one of these supplements, please check first with your healthcare practitioner for any interactions with existing medications or contraindications.

Chapter 4

Keeping the Heart Healthy

The loss of female sex hormones during the menopausal years has a marked impact on women's heart health. While menopause does not cause cardiovascular conditions, it does raise the risk for developing them. Hypertension (high blood pressure), which affects 26 per cent of women in the UK, and cardiovascular events remain the number-one cause of death in women post menopause.[1,2] In fact, high blood pressure (hypertension) increases the risk of arterial damage, promoting atherothrombosis and significantly raising the risk of ischemic stroke and cardiovascular events. As you approach menopause, make a point to regularly check your blood pressure, and take lifestyle and dietary measures to lower it if needed. Exercise, weight management and quality sleep are key lifestyle changes in addition to diet that can improve high blood pressure.

It is the decline in oestrogen in particular that contributes to changes in metabolic rate,[3] a shift to central adiposity (tummy fat), higher blood pressure and unfavourable changes in blood lipids (dyslipidemia).[4] Total cholesterol, low density lipoprotein (LDL) cholesterol and ApoB tend to rise during menopause.[5] (ApoB is one of the best markers for cardiovascular risk because each atherogenic lipoprotein particle – like LDL, VLDL, and Lp(a) – carries one ApoB molecule. That means ApoB levels strongly reflect the number of particles driving plaque formation, which is a better predictor of risk than LDL cholesterol alone.) One study found there was also a significant increase in the proportion of LDL cholesterol particles that were very small and dense, which are more strongly linked with an increased risk of heart disease – rising from 10 to 13 per cent in premenopausal women to 30 to 49 per cent after menopause.[6]

In addition, an immune shift that increases overall inflammation in the body further contributes to the heightened risk of cardiovascular issues during menopause.[7] Chronic inflammation irritates the blood vessels and contributes to the build-up of plaque. Over time, this plaque can become unstable, and when it ruptures, it can trigger the formation of blood clots, which may lead to heart attacks or strokes. Additional factors such as high blood pressure, high homocysteine, elevated LDL cholesterol and triglycerides, and increased ApoB – all of which may rise during the menopause transition can amplify this inflammatory response. This underlines the importance of a diet rich in antioxidant vitamins and polyphenols as well as heart-healthy omega-3 fatty acids and fibre. Metabolic changes, including increased insulin resistance and central fat accumulation, also play a role in sustaining chronic inflammation. The good news is that many of the menopause recipes included in this book focus on a more plant-rich Mediterranean style of eating, rich in nutrients known to support cardiovascular and metabolic health.

OESTROGEN AND THE HEART

There are numerous genes and enzymes regulated by oestrogen that are involved in heart health.[8] Some are involved in vasodilation and vasoconstriction,[9] immune activity, endothelial health, insulin sensitivity, clotting and lipid metabolism. In fact, oestrogen plays a key role in regulating inflammatory responses and supporting a healthy lipid profile. Oestrogen is also involved in the expression of genes for energy metabolism and mitochondrial health, which is equally important for healthy heart function and delivering energy to the body.[10] As oestrogen levels decline, the body faces a higher burden of oxidative stress, which can exacerbate inflammation and endothelial dysfunction. This makes incorporating antioxidant-rich, colourful plant foods into the diet even more important for heart health during menopause.

Nitric oxide production tends to decline with age and hormonal changes, particularly during menopause. Oestrogen supports nitric oxide production in endothelial cells.[11] Nitric oxide is a critical molecule for heart health due to its ability to promote vasodilation and support healthy blood pressure, maintain endothelial function, prevent atherosclerosis, regulate platelets, reduce inflammation and protect against ischaemia. Maintaining healthy levels of nitric oxide supports both heart health and healthy blood pressure. Certain foods rich in nitrates (found in rhubarb, leafy greens, beets and other vegetables) can support the body's production of nitric oxide (see box).

Of course, there are many other risk factors involved in heart health. Some are non-modifiable, such as age, genetic predisposition, race and family history. But there are many modifiable risk factors including diet, alcohol consumption, smoking, stress management, exercise and sleep. Note that certain underlying health conditions can also be associated with less favourable lipid measurements, such as thyroid disorders, kidney disease, liver disease and diabetes.

The menopause recipes in this book aim to address many of these modifiable factors by helping you maintain a healthy body composition (lose fat, improve muscle mass), improve insulin sensitivity, lower inflammation, improve lipid health and increase antioxidant capacity and nitric oxide levels.

You can see how menopause has a significant impact on heart health, but these changes start earlier than menopause. It is the perimenopause years, with fluctuating hormone levels, that are most often associated with heart palpitations, known as arrhythmia. Similarly, changes in sleep patterns or gradual weight gain during perimenopause can also impact heart health. Remember that carrying more abdominal fat is linked to insulin resistance and type 2 diabetes, which are risk factors for heart disease.

The gut–heart connection in menopause: Microbiome, metabolism, and cardiometabolic health

The gut microbiome plays a pivotal role in regulating oestrogen metabolism, lipid balance, inflammation, blood pressure and insulin sensitivity – all of which influence cardiometabolic health during menopause.

1. Gut microbiome and oestrogen metabolism

The gut houses bacteria that regulate oestrogen metabolism, collectively known as the *estrobolome* (see Chapter 11). These microbes influence oestrogen recycling through the production of *beta-glucuronidase*, an enzyme that deconjugates oestrogen in the gut, allowing it to be reabsorbed into circulation.

A balanced gut microbiome supports optimal oestrogen metabolism, which is critical for maintaining cardiovascular protection. When gut microbiome diversity declines – commonly observed during menopause – oestrogen metabolism can become disrupted, potentially reducing the recycling and bioavailability of oestrogen. Since oestrogen plays a protective role in vascular health, this dysregulation may contribute to an increased risk of heart disease.[12]

2. Impact on cholesterol and lipid metabolism

The gut microbiome plays a key role in lipid metabolism. Beneficial bacteria, such as *Lactobacillus* and *Bifidobacterium*, aid in breaking down dietary fats and reducing low-density lipoprotein (LDL) cholesterol levels through mechanisms such as bile acid metabolism and short-chain fatty acid (SCFA) production. Gut dysbiosis – an imbalance in microbial composition – can exacerbate lipid dysregulation.[13]

Menopause may contribute to this imbalance and increase systemic inflammation. A disrupted gut barrier, often seen with dysbiosis, can lead to increased intestinal permeability, allowing bacterial endotoxins like lipopolysaccharides (LPS) to enter the bloodstream. This, in turn, triggers chronic low-grade inflammation, a key driver of cardiovascular disease (CVD).[14]

Studies suggests that a diet rich in prebiotic fibre, polyphenols and probiotics can reduce systemic inflammation and improve gut barrier integrity.[15]

3. Blood pressure regulation

The gut microbiome plays a role in blood pressure regulation by producing SCFAs such as butyrate, acetate and propionate. These metabolites help modulate vascular tone, reduce arterial stiffness and improve endothelial function.[16]

Dysbiosis may impair SCFA production, contributing to hypertension.

4. Insulin sensitivity and metabolic health

Gut bacteria influence glucose metabolism and insulin sensitivity, both of which are critical for cardiovascular health. During menopause, there is an increased risk of insulin resistance, which contributes to weight gain, metabolic syndrome and elevated cardiovascular risk.

Targeted probiotic strains, such as *Lactobacillus rhamnosus* and *Bifidobacterium breve*, have demonstrated potential in improving metabolic health in postmenopausal women.[17]

For this reason, the menopause plan includes plenty of plant-based dishes, fermented foods, prebiotics and fibre.[18]

ROLE OF DIET AND HEART HEALTH

Diet can have a noticeable impact on heart health.[19] While dietary cholesterol has minimal effect on blood cholesterol levels for most people, high intakes of saturated fat – found in fatty cuts of meat, full-fat dairy, butter, and coconut oil – can in some people raise ApoB, a marker of the number of atherogenic lipoproteins, including LDL and VLDL. Research also points to ultra-processed foods – which are often high in added sugars, refined carbohydrates, and additives – as contributors to poor cardiovascular outcomes, partly through their impact on inflammation, insulin resistance, and lipid metabolism.[20] On the positive side, omega-3 fatty acids (found in oily fish like salmon and mackerel) can lower triglycerides, reduce blood pressure, and improve lipid profiles. Similarly, certain foods such as nuts and seeds, soy foods, foods rich in soluble fibre (oats, beans and pulses, seeds, certain fruits and vegetables) and plant sterols (e.g., nuts, seeds, wholegrains, fruits and vegetables, fortified foods) can all support healthy lipid levels. Garlic contains a plant compound called allicin, and diets rich in garlic may help reduce the risk of cardiovascular disease through lowering hypertension, promoting vasodilation, improving lipid levels and reducing the risk of plaque build-up in the arteries.[21]

The electrolytes particularly potassium and magnesium play a key role in supporting healthy blood pressure, while calcium from food sources may also contribute to blood pressure regulation and help promote a regular heartbeat. B vitamins play a key role in supporting the nervous system and may help protect against cardiovascular disease, stroke, and cognitive decline. Elevated levels of the amino acid homocysteine – which tend to rise with age – are linked to an increased risk of heart disease and cognitive issues. Vitamins B6, B9 (as folate or methylfolate), and B12 help reduce homocysteine levels and support vascular health. Additionally, thiamine (vitamin B1) contributes to normal heart function by supporting energy production in cardiac cells.

Incorporating phytoestrogenic rich foods can be beneficial for cardiovascular health. Some such as isoflavones (e.g., soy products) may improve blood lipids, endothelial function and reduce hypertension. They may also reduce arterial stiffness and oxidative stress.[22]

You will find the recipes in this book incorporate many key foods and nutrients associated with better cardiovascular health.

If you are concerned about supporting heart health, look for 'Heart health' on key recipes.

During menopause, hormonal changes significantly affects cardiometabolic health including lipid metabolism, insulin sensitivity, blood pressure regulation and vascular health. The following table highlights some of the key nutrients, their food sources, and how they support cardiometabolic health during this life stage. Many of these foods are included in the recipes and meal plans.

Table 4.1. Summary of heart health[23]

Category	Key nutrients	Example foods	Potential benefits
Lipid health	Omega-3 fatty acids	Fatty fish – salmon, sardines, mackerel (ALA found in flaxseeds, walnuts, chia seeds)	Anti-inflammatory, improves lipid profile
Lipid metabolism	Phytosterols	Nuts, seeds, soybeans, wheatgerm	Lowers LDL cholesterol and ApoB
	Polyphenols	Green tea, dark chocolate, berries, olives	Supports endothelial function, reduces oxidative stress

cont.

Category	Key nutrients	Example foods	Potential benefits
	Soluble fibre	Oats, beans and pulses, flaxseeds, apples, psyllium	Lowers LDL cholesterol, supports gut health
Vascular function and blood pressure	Nitrates	Beets, leafy greens, watermelon	Supports healthy blood pressure, platelet aggregation control, endothelial function, myocardial function
	Magnesium	Nuts, seeds, leafy greens, seafood	Regulates blood pressure, supports vascular health, improves insulin sensitivity
	Vitamin C and polyphenols	Citrus, berries, green tea, dark chocolate, olives	Antioxidant, enhances nitric oxide production, protects NO from oxidative degradation, and improves endothelial function
	Sulphur compounds	Garlic, onions, leeks	Supports nitric oxide production and healthy blood pressure, reduces oxidative stress
	Phytoestrogens (isoflavones, lignans)	Soy products (tofu, tempeh, soy milk), flaxseeds, sesame seeds, chickpeas	Enhances vascular function and lipid profile via oestrogen receptor modulation and nitric oxide support
Homocysteine and cardiovascular risk	B6, B12, folate	Leafy greens, eggs, poultry, fish	Reduces homocysteine, lowers cardiovascular risk
Metabolic health and insulin sensitivity (see also Chapter 3)	Resveratrol	Red grapes, berries, peanuts	Enhances insulin sensitivity and glucose uptake in muscle and adipose tissue
	Alpha-lipoic acid	Organ meats, spinach (ALA, also as supplement)	Reduces inflammation, improves insulin sensitivity

	Prebiotic fibre and probiotics	Garlic, onions, asparagus, fermented foods (e.g. kefir, yogurt, kimchi)	Supports microbiome balance, regulates blood sugar
Antioxidant and anti-inflammatory support	Coenzyme Q10 (CoQ10)	Organ meats, fatty fish, spinach, nuts	Supports heart mitochondrial function, reduces oxidative stress
Arterial health	Vitamin K2 (MK-7)	Natto, aged cheese, egg yolks, butter from grass-fed cows	Prevents arterial calcification, supports bone and heart health

Dietary nitrates for heart health

Nitric oxide is produced naturally by the body and it is vital for our health. It helps regulate blood pressure, maintains endothelial health and has important anti-inflammatory and antioxidant effects making it cardioprotective. However, levels of nitric oxide decline as we age, and particularly post menopause. Oestrogen supports the expression and activation of eNOS, which is endothelial nitric oxide synthase, an enzyme found in the endothelium (the inner lining of blood vessels). eNOS produces nitric oxide (NO) – a gas that helps blood vessels relax and widen (a process called vasodilation). Nitric oxide also helps reduce inflammation, prevents blood clotting, and protects against atherosclerosis (plaque build-up in arteries). So when oestrogen declines around menopause, this protective mechanism weakens. As a result, nitric oxide production decreases, leading to stiffer blood vessels, increased inflammation, and a greater risk of developing cardiovascular diseases such as hypertension and atherosclerosis. This is one of the reasons why the risk of heart disease rises significantly in women after menopause. We can support the production of nitric oxide by consuming nitrate-rich vegetables, which naturally contain antioxidants and polyphenols that enhance the conversion of nitrate to nitric oxide while also protecting against oxidative stress. These nitrates are reduced to nitrite and then to nitric oxide by commensal bacteria in the mouth.

This is why protecting the oral and gut microbiome, which convert nitrate into nitric oxide, is so important. It is also helpful to avoid indiscriminate mouthwash use that disrupts this conversion.[24] Daily intake of nitrate-rich foods, such as beetroot juice, has been shown to lower inflammation, improve the function of the endothelium (the cells that line the inside of all blood vessels) and improve circulation. This is beneficial not just to the heart but also to other areas of the body, including brain function.[25]

There are many nitrate-rich foods, although most studies have been undertaken using beetroot juice. Nitrate-rich vegetables include: beetroot (especially beetroot juice), leafy greens (kale, spinach, Swiss chard, mustard greens), radishes, rhubarb, celery, carrots, red and green cabbage, parsley and coriander. The menopause plan incorporates many of these nitrate-rich foods.

Chapter 5

Optimizing Brain Function

Ovarian hormones are crucial for brain health and influence many aspects of cognition, memory and mood. In fact, having and maintaining physiological levels of testosterone, progesterone and oestrogen is important for optimal brain health and function. We have receptors for sex hormones distributed throughout the brain as well as being found in the mitochondria. So important are these hormones (and their derivatives) to the brain that the brain is capable of producing its own via cholesterol and from the conversion of peripheral blood steroid hormones into derivatives (e.g., conversion of testosterone to oestradiol via the activity of the enzyme aromatase).

COGNITIVE HEALTH

Oestrogen is critical to proper brain function, including cognition and mood.[1] Oestradiol is important for neural plasticity[2] and may influence neurogenesis in the hippocampus (neurogenesis refers to the process of generating new neurons, or nerve cells, in the brain). The hippocampus is a region within the brain that is particularly important for learning and memory processes. Having optimal levels of oestradiol therefore plays a key role in supporting learning and memory.[3]

The brain also responds to circulating oestrogen, which crosses the blood–brain barrier. As levels of sex hormones decline throughout the body at menopause, this has an impact on overall levels in the brain.

The dominant form of oestrogen post menopause is oestrone, which, unlike oestradiol, has not been shown to have these beneficial effects on the brain. The profound effect of oestradiol in the brain has led to investigations into the potential benefits of using bioidentical HRT for brain health and function.[4]

The brain, despite accounting for only 2 per cent of the body's weight, consumes at least 20 per cent of the body's fuel for energy production. Any decline in mitochondrial function or energy delivery to the brain can lead to cognitive impairments, affecting both mood and cognition. Oestrogen has beneficial effects on brain energy metabolism by increasing blood flow, delivering nutrients to the brain and facilitating glucose uptake and energy (ATP, adenosine triphosphate) production. Oestrogen influences glucose transport in the brain through multiple glucose transporters (e.g., GLUT1, GLUT3, GLUT4).

Beyond glucose transport, oestrogen plays a key role in mitochondrial health and function.[5] It promotes mitochondrial biogenesis (the formation of new mitochondria) and helps eliminate damaged mitochondria through apoptosis (programmed cell death). The loss of oestrogen during menopause can disrupt these processes, impairing brain metabolism and mitochondrial function.[6] Since many aspects of brain ageing, cognitive decline and neurodegenerative diseases such as Alzheimer's and Parkinson's are related to mitochondrial dysfunction, these effects are particularly relevant to brain health during menopause. Supporting mitochondria through diet and lifestyle can help maintain cognitive health (see Table 5.1.).

One of the notable effects of oestradiol in the brain is its ability to increase the expression of brain-derived neurotrophic factor (BDNF) and activate its receptor. BDNF and oestrogen appear to work together to support neuron growth, survival, neural plasticity and learning. BDNF plays a crucial role in overall brain health, cognition and mood, so you want to maintain optimal levels of BDNF. The problem is that BDNF, like oestrogen, drops significantly after menopause (see box).

Sex hormones, particularly oestrogen, are also neuroprotective – that is, they possess antioxidant properties to protect neurons from damage.[7] Fluctuations in oestrogen levels, particularly during the menopause transition, can affect vulnerability to neurological disorders.[8] Oestrogen also impacts neuroinflammation. In fact, a key role of oestrogen is its influence on controlling inflammation. Both ageing and menopause cause a dysregulation in various immune cells, which, in turn, lead to increased neuroinflammation. This link with oestrogen and menopause may explain why studies suggest that women have significant increases in inflammation in many areas of the brain compared to men as they age. This may in part explain why menopausal women have a higher prevalence and greater severity of Alzheimer's disease than men.[9, 10]

Another way oestrogen influences the brain during menopause is through its effect on the cholinergic system, a network in the brain associated with the neurotransmitter acetylcholine, which plays a key role in memory, learning and attention. In fact, the basal forebrain cholinergic systems, a specific part of the cholinergic system in the brain, requires the presence of oestrogen to function properly. Lower oestrogen levels around menopause[11] increase the importance of getting sufficient choline, a nutrient that the body converts into acetylcholine.[12] For these reasons, including foods to support the production of acetylcholine (including choline-rich foods) becomes particularly important around menopause (see box).

Brain fog and neuroinflammation

Brain fog is a common symptom experienced during perimenopause and menopause, and can be quite alarming, such as suddenly forgetting the names of colleagues or losing track of what you were planning to do. For others, it just feels like you are struggling to focus or concentrate on tasks. There are many contributing factors to brain fog, but central is the decline in oestrogen levels and neuroinflammation. In fact, low-grade inflammation has been shown to impact both attention and cognition.[13] It's also worth checking thyroid function, as underactive thyroid (hypothyroidism) can mimic or exacerbate symptoms of brain fog and fatigue, particularly during midlife.

If you experience heavier bleeds during perimenopause (which can occur due to changes in the balance between oestrogen and progesterone) or are following a vegan or more plant-based diet, you may wish to check your iron status. This can impact oxygenation in the body and brain, which can contribute to a foggy head and fatigue. Focus on including iron-rich foods daily such as lean meat, poultry, fish, legumes, dark leafy greens, tempeh and natto, nuts and seeds (pumpkin seeds, sunflower seeds, almonds), quinoa, dried fruits (apricots, raisins, prunes). For better absorption of plant-based, non-heme iron, it's helpful to pair these with vitamin C-rich foods, such as citrus fruits, bell peppers, berries and leafy greens. This can significantly enhance the bioavailability of the iron from plant sources.

Hydration and electrolyte balance are also important, and often over-looked, contributors to cognitive clarity. Oestrogen helps regulate fluid balance and electrolyte retention, so its decline during menopause can alter thirst perception and kidney function, increasing the risk of mild dehydration. Even a 1–2% drop in hydration can impair attention, memory and mood. Electrolytes like sodium, potassium and magnesium are essential for nerve signaling and brain cell communication, and imbalances may contribute to symptoms of brain fog. Supporting hydration with regular water intake and including electrolyte-rich foods – such as leafy greens, bananas, nuts, seeds and legumes – may help support mental clarity.[14]

The reduction in the neurotransmitter acetylcholine may also play a role, emphasizing the importance of consuming sufficient choline-rich foods in the diet. Maintaining a diverse gut microbiome is essential for mitigating neuroinflammation, as the gut–brain axis plays a critical role in immune regulation and neurological health. A diet rich in dietary fibre, prebiotics and polyphenols – found in a variety of colourful plant foods – supports microbial diversity and short-chain fatty acid (SCFA) production, which have anti-inflammatory effects. Additionally, consuming fermented foods such as kefir, yogurt and kimchi provides probiotics that enhance gut barrier integrity and modulate immune responses. This not only supports gastrointestinal function but also contributes to reducing systemic and neuroinflammation, ultimately benefiting cognitive function and overall brain health.

Dietary changes aimed at addressing neuroinflammation, mitochon-drial dysfunction and hormonal shifts can help reduce cognitive issue, brain fog and long-term neurodegenerative risks.

Table 5.1. Key foods and nutrients supporting
cognitive health during menopause

Category	Key nutrients/ compounds	Example foods	Potential benefits
Mitochondrial and energy support	Coenzyme Q10	Small amounts in fatty fish, organ meats, nuts, spinach, broccoli (mainly via supplementation)	Supports mitochondrial function, combats oxidative stress
	Creatine	Red meat, poultry, fish	Helps energy production, supports cognitive function
	L-carnitine	Red meat, dairy, fish, poultry	Enhances energy production in brain cells, reduces mental fatigue, protects against oxidative stress
	Electrolytes, including sodium, potassium, calcium and magnesium	Fruits and vegetables, dairy, sea salt, nuts, seeds	Support brain function during stress, regulate brain electrical activity
	Iron	Red meat, poultry, legumes, leafy greens, fish and shellfish	Essential for oxygen transport and energy production
Anti-inflammatory and antioxidant support	Curcumin	Turmeric + black pepper and fat for absorption (mainly via supplementation)	Reduces brain inflammation
	Polyphenols such as resveratrol, quercetin, EGCG	Berries, grapes (resveratrol), green tea (EGCG), onions, apples	Lower inflammation and oxidative stress, enhance cognitive function, protect against age-related cognitive decline
	NAC/glutathione	Supports production of glutathione: garlic, onions, cruciferous vegetables (e.g., broccoli, cabbage), spinach, avocados, whey protein (mainly via supplementation)	Reduces oxidative stress, lowers inflammation, supports cognitive function and mitochondrial function

cont.

Category	Key nutrients/ compounds	Example foods	Potential benefits
Methylation and cognition (see also BDNF, page 58)	B vitamins (B1, B2, B3, B5, B6, B12, Folate)	Eggs, dairy, fish, leafy greens, legumes	Support energy metabolism and cognition, lower homocysteine levels (B6, B12, folate)
	Zinc and selenium	Seafood, Brazil nuts, pumpkin seeds	Support neurotransmitter activity, neuroprotective, thyroid health
	Omega-3 fatty acids (EPA and DHA)	Fatty fish (e.g., salmon, sardines, mackerel)	Essential for brain structure, mood and memory
	Choline	Eggs, liver, soybeans, fish, poultry	Supports acetylcholine production, memory, and brain cell membrane structure
	Phosphatidylserine	Soy, fish, organ meats, eggs	Supports brain cell membranes and cognitive function
	Phytoestrogens	Soy, flaxseeds, chickpeas, lentils	Mild oestrogenic effect, neuroprotective, supports cognition
Blood sugar and gut–brain axis (see also Chapter 2)	Fibre and prebiotics	Fruits and vegetables, legumes, whole grains, nuts, seeds	Balance blood sugar, support gut–brain axis and oestrogen metabolism
	Probiotics	Yogurt, kefir, kimchi, sauerkraut	Support gut–brain axis, modulate inflammation
	Magnesium	Leafy greens, nuts, seeds, legumes, whole grains	Lowers stress, aids sleep, improves insulin sensitivity, helps to stabilize blood sugar levels

Foods to support acetylcholine production

Acetylcholine is a neurotransmitter involved in numerous physiological processes but particularly important for memory, learning and cognition. Here are some key foods to support acetylcholine production:

- *Choline-rich foods:* Choline is a key precursor for acetylcholine synthesis and found in:
    - egg yolks
    - organ meats (such as liver, kidney)
    - fish (e.g., cod, salmon)
    - poultry (chicken, turkey)
    - dairy products (e.g., milk, yogurt)
    - soy products (e.g., edamame beans, tofu)
    - nuts (especially peanuts)
    - cruciferous vegetables (e.g., broccoli, cauliflower, Brussels sprouts).

- *B vitamins:* Certain B vitamins – particularly B6, B12 and folate – are involved in the metabolism of choline and can indirectly support acetylcholine production. Good food sources include:
    - wholegrains (e.g., brown rice, oats, quinoa)
    - leafy green vegetables (e.g., spinach, kale)
    - nuts and seeds
    - lean meats and poultry
    - dairy products (e.g., milk, yogurt)
    - legumes (e.g., beans, lentils).

- *Omega-3 fatty acids:* These are important for brain health and may support the release of acetylcholine. Sources of omega-3 fatty acids include:
    - fatty fish (e.g., salmon, mackerel, sardines), rich in omega-3, particularly EPA and DHA, which are beneficial for brain function
    - flaxseeds and flaxseed oil – plant-based sources of ALA

(alpha-linolenic acid), which the body can partially convert to EPA and DHA
- walnuts – source of ALA
- chia seeds – source of ALA.

- *Antioxidants:* Antioxidants can help protect cholinergic neurons and maintain their function. Foods rich in antioxidants include:
  - berries and super berry powders like acai
  - dark chocolate and raw cacao
  - green tea/matcha green tea powder
  - spinach and other leafy greens
  - nuts and seeds.

- *Herbs and spices:* Some herbs and spices may have compounds that support brain health and cholinergic function. These include:
  - turmeric (curcumin)
  - rosemary
  - sage.

HORMONES AND MOOD

Many women experience mood changes during menopause, including mood swings, irritability and anxiety, and even symptoms of depression. In fact, depressive symptoms increase two to four times as women transition through menopause.[15]

These changes may, in part, be related to the decline in oestrogen levels and its influence on serotonin and dopamine pathways. Dopamine is a neurotransmitter associated with various functions, including mood regulation, reward processing and cognitive function. Oestrogen has been shown to modulate dopamine activity in the brain influencing dopamine availability, receptor density and the activity of dopamine transporters. The decrease in oestrogen levels during menopause may therefore indirectly affect dopamine function and increase the risk of low mood and reduced motivation.[16]

Serotonin, which is often referred to as a mood-boosting neurotrans-mitter, is also influenced by oestrogen levels. Oestrogen affects the avail-ability and activity of serotonin in the brain. The loss of oestrogen at menopause results in decreased density of certain serotonin receptors, known as 5-HT2A receptors, and a lower activity of serotonin. In addition, these 5-HT2A receptors in the central nervous system are responsible for temperature regulation and may play a role in hot flashes and night sweats.[17] Fluctuations in oestrogen around perimenopause can also lead to changes in serotonin, in turn increasing vasodilation in the brain, which can be linked to headaches. But one of the profound effects of reduced serotonin levels is low mood[18] and an increased risk of depression.

To support serotonin levels, pay attention to both foods and nutrients that can improve BDNF as well as serotonin specifically (see box). The production of serotonin requires the amino acid L-tryptophan (found in foods such as oats, bananas, dried prunes, milk, fish, cheese, chicken, turkey, peanuts and chocolate). A number of vitamins and minerals are also required for serotonin production including iron, B6, methyl B12, methylfolate, magnesium and vitamin D. Also pay attention to blood sugar levels and ensuring sufficient omega-3-rich foods in the diet. Supplements such as 5-HTP (a precursor of serotonin) and the nutrient inositol can be useful to help improve serotonin levels (inositol improves sensitivity of serotonin receptors). (Note that 5-HTP should not be taken if you are on antidepressants.)

There are several ways to support dopamine levels. First, ensure you are consuming sufficient protein-rich foods at each meal to provide plenty of the amino acid L-tyrosine (good foods include meat, nuts, avocado, eggs, yogurt, beans, fish and chicken) and phenylalanine (found in meat, poultry, egg, soy, fish, nuts and seeds). Various vitamins and minerals are required for the production of dopamine, particularly B6, zinc, mag-nesium and methylfolate. Other foods and nutrients, such as L-theanine (found in green tea), omega-3 fatty acids and the adaptogenic herb rhod-iola can support dopamine levels while choline may enhance the release of dopamine.

Managing stress, getting sufficient quality sleep, exercising daily and building strong supportive connections with others are all important when it comes to managing mood (see Part 3). Some studies have also found that acupuncture[19] can alter neurotransmitters in the brain to alleviate conditions such as anxiety and nervousness, improving overall mood.

It is not just oestrogen that influences brain health, cognition and mood. Progesterone also plays a key role in modulating neuroinflammation and may have a protective effect on myelin, the fatty substance that forms an insulating sheath around nerve fibres (axons) in the nervous system.[20] When myelin is damaged, as seen in conditions like multiple sclerosis (MS), it can lead to neurological symptoms, including mood disturbances. Impaired myelin can disrupt communication between brain areas that regulate emotions, cognition and behaviour. Therefore, the protection and repair of myelin are essential for maintaining healthy brain function and emotional balance.

Additionally, chronic or excessive neuroinflammation can negatively impact brain function and is linked to several mood disorders, such as anxiety and depression. Inflammatory cytokines, small proteins involved in immune responses, can interfere with normal neurotransmitter activity and neural communication, leading to changes in mood and behaviour. Progesterone appears to play a direct role in cognition and mood regulation.[21] Low levels of progesterone can contribute to symptoms like anxiety, irritability, depression and sleep disturbances.

Testosterone also impacts cognition and mood in women. Studies suggest that testosterone has anti-anxiety and anti-depressive effects.[22,23] Testosterone also affects processes like neurogenesis and the development of neurons in various brain regions, including the hippocampus (linked to learning and memory), making it equally important for overall cognition.[24]

If you are looking to optimize brain health and cognition through the menopause and beyond, look for 'Brain health' on key recipes.

SUPPORTING BRAIN-DERIVED NEUROTROPHIC FACTOR

BDNF (Brain-Derived Neurotrophic Factor) is both a growth factor and a protein and plays a crucial role in learning and cognition. BDNF is a key regulator of synaptic plasticity, which is the brain's ability to change and adapt in response to experiences and learning. It enhances the formation and strengthening of synapses, making it easier for neurons to communicate with each other. This synaptic plasticity is fundamental for learning and memory processes. BDNF supports the generation of new neurons in the hippocampus, a brain region critical for learning and memory. The production of new neurons (neurogenesis) is associated with improved memory formation and cognitive flexibility. Elevated levels of BDNF have been linked to improved memory formation and retention. Levels of BDNF decline with age, but more significantly around menopause, which could, in turn, impact brain health, cognition and mood.

Six lifestyle practices that boost BDNF

- *Exercise:* Both aerobic exercise (e.g., jogging, swimming, cycling and brisk walking) and strength training exercises can increase levels of BDNF.

- *Sun exposure:* BDNF levels rise and fall with the seasons – they are naturally higher during spring and summer but lower in the autumn and winter. This is related to the production of vitamin D, which can influence BDNF levels. Try to get outside each day, even if it's only for a 10-minute stroll around your block, to get a bit of sunshine on your skin.

- *Quality sleep:* Deep sleep is beneficial because it helps you rest and repair. Deep, restorative sleep, especially during the later stages of the sleep cycle, is when your body naturally releases more BDNF.

- *Stress management:* Chronic stress can reduce BDNF levels. Practising stress-reduction techniques such as mindfulness meditation, deep breathing exercises or yoga can help (see Chapter 9).

- *Learning and mental stimulation:* Continuous learning and challenging your brain through activities such as puzzles, learning a new language or acquiring new skills can promote BDNF production.

Key foods that increase BDNF

- *Fatty fish:* Fatty fish such as salmon, mackerel and trout are rich in omega-3 fatty acids, particularly docosahexaenoic acid (DHA), which has been shown to increase BDNF levels.

- *Curcumin (turmeric):* Curcumin, the active compound in turmeric, has demonstrated neuroprotective and anti-inflammatory properties. The polyphenols in this spice increase BDNF levels. Curcumin bioavailability is limited from food sources. If you choose to add turmeric to your food or beverages, make sure to pair it with black pepper and a fat source. These both improve the amount that your body absorbs.

- *Blueberries:* Blueberries are high in antioxidants and polyphenols, which may have neuroprotective effects and support cognitive health as well as increase BDNF.[25]

- *Matcha green tea:* Green tea contains compounds like catechins and L-theanine, which may have cognitive-enhancing properties. It has been associated with improved cognitive function and attention.

- *Dark chocolate:* Cacao contains the phytonutrients that increase BDNF. Ideally, choose a dark 85–100 per cent cacao chocolate for higher antioxidant levels.

- *Coffee:* Moderate coffee consumption (about 1–3 cups per day) has been associated with improved cognitive function and a potential increase in BDNF levels due to caffeine content. Be mindful of your tolerance as too much can impact stress hormones and sleep.

- *Eggs:* The omega-3 content of eggs has been linked to higher BDNF levels. The eggs with the best omega-3 profile are often from pasture-raised chickens.[26]

- *Soy:* Organic whole and fermented soy products[27] such as tempeh are associated with neuroprotection, possibly through BDNF increase.

- *Extra virgin olive oil (EVOO):* Go for cold-pressed, extra-virgin olive oil, which is higher in phenolic compounds. EVOO[28] consumption has been associated with improvements in mood and increases in expression of BDNF.

- *Red grapes:* Organic dark-coloured grapes[29] are a good source of resveratrol and other polyphenols like flavonoids, which have also been linked to improved cognitive health. These compounds may work synergistically to support overall brain function and potentially increase BDNF levels.

- *Lion's Mane mushrooms (Hericium erinaceus)* may stimulate the production of BDNF, supporting brain health and cognitive function.[30]

Chapter 6

Bone Health

Woman can lose up to 20 per cent of their bone density during the five to seven years following menopause. While there are a number of factors involved in supporting bone health, it is evident that reduced hormone production, particularly oestrogen, causes changes in various biochemical pathways that lead to increased bone loss.

Bones are living organs that are constantly remodelling throughout our lives. In optimal bone health, an equilibrium is maintained between bone disintegration (bone resorption) and bone formation. As we age, this balance shifts, increasing the rate of bone loss. In menopausal women, this rate of bone loss is more evident due to hormone decline and an increase in inflammatory signals in the body.[1] Low bone density increases the risk for bone fracture. Osteoporosis is often referred to as a silent disease because there are few symptoms. Many women only find out they have a problem with their bone density after a fall.

The reduction in oestrogen in particular results in an increase in bone resorption leading to bone loss and microfractures. Oestrogen and calcium also have a relationship when it comes to bone health. Oestrogen supports intestinal absorption of calcium. So, having low oestrogen levels can negatively impact the amount of calcium you're able to absorb. This is one of the reasons why ensuring sufficient calcium intake is important around menopause. Progesterone, like oestrogen, plays an important role in bone turnover and bone formation, while testosterone plays a key role in bone formation. In view of the important role hormones play in supporting bone health, if you are concerned about your bone health, speak to your healthcare practitioner regarding the use of bioidentical hormones.

Stress and sleep can also impact bone health. When your body is stressed, it releases a steroid hormone called cortisol. Cortisol indirectly acts on bone by blocking calcium absorption, which decreases bone cell growth. Stress increases the rate at which your body uses magnesium, which is another key mineral for bone health. Chronic stress can also have an inflammatory effect on the body, and it is now evident that one of the key drivers for bone loss is low-grade inflammation. Following a Mediterranean style of eating, with plenty of fruits, vegetables, nuts, seeds, monounsaturated fats, omega-3 fats from oily fish, fermented foods and sufficient protein can help provide the essential nutrients for bone health while keeping inflammation in check.

Stress and, of course, menopause itself can also impact sleep patterns. Bone turnover markers (BTMs) increase overnight and peak in the early morning, and then decrease as the day progresses. Disruption in your sleep may cause dysregulation of the bone formation process.[2] In other words, if you aren't sleeping soundly overnight, it may disturb your bone cells' genetic expression for remodelling.[3]

Exercise[4] plays an important role in maintaining bone health. Exercise stimulates osteogenesis, the development and formation of bones.[5] Weight-bearing and resistance exercise is particularly useful for helping to maintain bone health and improving bone mineral density.[6] Exercise not only improves muscle strength, balance and fitness, but also reduces the incidence of falls and fractures. Resistance/weight-bearing exercises are particularly beneficial, especially when targeted exercises are performed on key areas of the body and with progressive overload, where the weight is gradually increased over time.[7] Include compound, multi-joint exercises (e.g., squats, deadlifts, bench press). Ideally aim for at least 3–4 days per week of strength training. For noticeable improvements, exercise needs to be undertaken consistently over a long period of time (at least 6–9 months).[8] Please note that if you have been diagnosed with osteoporosis, work with a qualified fitness instructor who can advise on the most appropriate exercises.

DIETARY FACTORS

When it comes to diet, there are a wealth of key nutrients required for optimal bone health.

Collagen is the body's most abundant structural protein, meaning it acts like the glue that holds your body together. Bones are made up of about 35 per cent collagen.[9] It provides a framework for the bones and, along with calcium and other nutrients, strengthens them. The problem is that as we age, our ability to produce collagen rapidly declines. By the age of 25, collagen production is already declining. After your 50s, over 15 per cent of the body's production capacity will be gone. And after age 70, over 30 per cent of collagen is completely lost. While collagen is naturally produced by the body, this significant decline makes it difficult to rely on the body's own capacity to produce it, which is why supplementation may be beneficial. Research has shown certain types of bioactive collagen peptides can lead to improvements in bone density.[10] As vitamin C is crucial for supporting collagen production, you should also focus on increasing the variety of fruits and vegetables in your diet.

Protein is a key macronutrient for bone health.[11] Research shows that protein may support your bones in several ways, including parathyroid regulation and enhancing calcium absorption.[12] A diet rich in protein (1.5–2 g/kg body weight/day) decreases the risk of fractures.[13]

As inflammation is a driver in bone loss, following a diet known for its anti-inflammatory benefits, such as the Mediterranean style of eating, may be helpful. This type of eating is plant heavy, with plenty of herbs and spices, fermented foods, monounsaturated fats and omega-3 fatty acids, as well as sufficient protein. The recipes in this book are designed with these key elements in mind.

A wide range of vitamins and minerals are important for supporting a healthy bone matrix, and some of the key nutrients are highlighted in Table 6.1. However, it is also important to consider the broader context of bone health around menopause, including the roles of chronic low-grade inflammation, hormonal changes and emerging evidence on the gut–bone axis. These are also included in the table.

Table 6.1. Nutrients to support bone health during menopause

Nutrient	Food sources	Action
Bone Matrix Support		
Calcium	Dairy products, calcium-set tofu, fortified plant-based milks and yogurts, leafy greens like kale and pak choi, nuts and seeds (especially almonds and sesame), tempeh, dried figs	Key mineral for bone matrix – 99% of calcium in your body is in your bones and teeth. Postmenopausal women at risk of osteoporosis are recommended to consume from food and supplements (if needed) combined 1000–1200 mg/day. The bioavailability of calcium supplements varies. Forms like microcrystalline hydroxyapatite (MCHA) and calcium citrate may have superior absorption.
Magnesium	Sesame seeds, almonds, dark chocolate, black beans, leafy greens	Supports osteoblast (bone-forming cell) activity. Regulates osteoclast (bone-resorbing cell) activity, helping maintain bone remodeling balance. Aids calcium absorption and bone mineralization.
Vitamin D	Mushrooms, oily fish, prawns, egg yolks, fortified foods, fortified milk alternatives	Essential for calcium and phosphorus utilization, supporting bone mineralization and overall bone health.
Boron	Dried fruits, peanut butter, nuts, lentils, chickpeas, kidney beans	Improves calcium and magnesium absorption and enhances vitamin D activity.
Copper	Oysters, kale, shiitake mushrooms, prunes	Works with enzymes like lysyl oxidase to incorporate collagen and elastin into the bone matrix.
Manganese	Mussels, hazelnuts, pumpkin seeds, wholegrains	Essential for bone formation and mineralization.
Phosphorous	Salmon, lean beef, Brazil nuts, lentils	85% of phosphorus is in bones, where it works with calcium and magnesium to form and maintain the bone matrix.
Potassium	Fruits and vegetables, especially bananas, butternut/acorn squash, potatoes	Reduces urinary calcium loss, helping to conserve calcium in the body to support bone density.
Silica/silicon	Leeks, beans, strawberries, rhubarb, horsetail	Supports collagen formation, important for bone strength and mineralization.

cont.

Nutrient	Food sources	Action
Bone Matrix Support		
Vitamin K2	Natto, certain hard cheeses and egg yolks. Vitamin K1 (which can be converted to K2 in the gut) is found in leafy greens, peas, blueberries, asparagus, broccoli and Brussels sprouts	Activates proteins responsible for delivering calcium to the bones (osteocalcin) and preventing calcium from depositing in soft tissues, like arteries, heart or kidneys.
Zinc	Seafood, spinach, red meat, seeds, nuts	Supports osteoblast activity and is involved in bone formation, repair and maintaining bone density.
Creatine	Animal foods (meat, fish, seafood)	Creatine supplementation may enhance osteoblast activity, promoting bone formation. This is partly due to creatine's role in increasing muscle mass and strength, as greater muscle mass can lead to increased mechanical loading on bones, which, in turn, stimulates bone formation and osteoblast activity.
B Vitamins	**B2 (Riboflavin):** Spinach, beet greens, mushrooms, almonds, dairy **B3 (Niacin):** Tuna, poultry, wild salmon **B6:** Turkey, beef, sweet potatoes, sunflower seeds, bananas **B9 (Folate):** Asparagus, beans, spinach, eggs **B12:** meat, seafood, dairy, eggs (animal sources only)	Enhance blood flow and nutrient delivery to bone (B3). Improve magnesium absorption (B6). Facilitate methylation and folate cycles (B6, B9, B12), essential for DNA repair and cell replication in bone tissue. Help with the synthesis of glutathione, a key protective antioxidant. Regulate homocysteine levels (B6, B9, B12); elevated homocysteine is associated with bone fragility.
Collagen	Bone broth, chicken skin, fish skin, pork skin, collagen supplements	Provides structural support to bones, helping maintain their strength and flexibility. Supports bone mineralization and the function of osteoblasts (bone-building cells).
Protein	Lean meats, fish, eggs, dairy, legumes, tofu, lentils	Helps in the formation and repair of bone tissue, promotes collagen production, and contributes to overall bone density by supporting osteoblast function.

Antioxidant and Anti-inflammatory Action		
Omega 3 DHA and EPA	Oily fish (sardines, mackerel, anchovies, salmon)	By reducing inflammation, EPA and DHA help lower osteoclast activity. These omega-3s promote osteoblast activity, which supports the formation of new bone.
Vitamin C	Citrus, berries, kiwifruit, bell peppers, dark leafy greens	Lowers inflammation, antioxidant protection, supports synthesis of the glutathione, promotes collagen formation.
Vitamin E	Nuts and seeds, brown rice, oats	Protects against free radical damage, which otherwise increases osteoclast activity, lowers inflammation.
Coenzyme Q10	Organ Meats, fatty fish (limited in food sources)	Antioxidant, promotes osteoblast differentiation and proliferation and matrix mineralization.
Curcumin	Turmeric (limited in food sources)	Antioxidant and anti-inflammatory properties, promotes osteoblast proliferation and differentiation, and regulates osteoblast and osteoclast formation.
Phytoestrogens	Isoflavones (tofu, tempeh, edamame, soy milk, miso, soy protein) Lignans (flaxseed, sesame seed)	Mimic oestrogen enhancing bone formation, improves bone mineralization, improves bone mineral density, reduces oxidative stress.
Selenium	Sunflower seeds, shellfish, poultry, eggs	Reduces oxidative stress, supporting bone and joint health by protecting bone cells from damage.
Gut-Bone Axis		
Fermented Foods	Fermented foods (yogurt, kefir, sauerkraut, kimchi)	Probiotic bacteria support bone density by improving mineral absorption and modulating immune response, reducing inflammation. Modulation of oestrogen metabolism (estrobolome activity).
Fibre / Prebiotics	**Resistant Starch:** (e.g. green bananas, plantains, cooked and cooled potatoes, cooked and cooled rice) **Fibre:** wholegrains, fruit, vegetables, legumes	Production of short-chain fatty acids (SCFAs), especially butyrate, which enhances bone mineralization and promote bone matrix formation, lowers inflammation, regulates osteoblast and osteoclast activity.

Lowering inflammation

Other nutrients have also been found to be important for bone health – antioxidants such as vitamins C and E, for example, help to counter the effects of oxidative stress on bone, which, when in excess, can shift the bone remodelling process, increasing bone loss. Curcumin (found in turmeric) has a variety of functions that can benefit bone health including antioxidant and anti-inflammatory properties. Studies have shown curcumin positively regulates the differentiation and promotes the proliferation of osteoblasts, which play a crucial role in bone formation. Multiple studies have shown that curcumin is effective in the treatment of osteoporosis as it interacts with a variety of signalling pathway targets, thereby interfering with the formation of osteoblasts and osteoclasts and regulating the development of osteoporosis.[14]

Omega-3 fatty acids are equally beneficial. These essential fats are known for their anti-inflammatory properties, particularly EPA (eicosapentaenoic acid) and DHA (docosahexaenoic acid). When inflammatory chemicals are high, it increases the activity of osteoclast cells (the cells that break down bone), which is why inflammation is so detrimental to bone health. By lowering inflammation, EPA and DHA help reduce osteoclast activity. At the same time, studies show that EPA and DHA can increase the activity of osteoblasts – the cells responsible for building new bone. Oily fish (sardines, mackerel, trout, salmon, etc.) is one of the best food sources of EPA and DHA.

The gut microbiome has also been shown to impact bone health. Certain probiotic bacteria, for example, appear to improve bone density, which may, in part, be due to their action on increasing mineral absorption and modulating the immune response, lowering inflammation. Sufficient fibre and prebiotics in the diet can support the production of SCFAs like butyrate, which also appear to have a beneficial effect on bone health.

Certain phytoestrogens appear to beneficial. Some, such as those found in soy products, may impact calcium metabolism and directly influence bone metabolism by binding to oestrogen receptors. Including these in your diet may be helpful (see Chapter 11).

If you are looking to support bone and joint health, look for 'Bone health' on key recipes.

PART 3

IMPORTANCE OF LIFESTYLE

Lifestyle factors like sleep, stress management and exercise are not only fundamental to navigating the challenges of menopause; they also play a key role in promoting long-term wellbeing and overall health. The following chapters address three essential elements – movement and exercise, sleep and stress management.

Chapter 7

Movement and Exercise

Regular exercise is immensely important for both physical and mental health at any age. In fact, exercise is probably one of the most potent longevity aids. It can support cardiometabolic health, muscle mass, joint and bone health, and even mental health. Studies have also shown it may help alleviate some of the symptoms commonly associated with menopause.[1]

Building in a comprehensive exercise programme during the perimenopause and menopause years is one of the most powerful tools for combating age-related loss in muscle mass, supporting bone density and improving overall health in the long term. The earlier you start to prioritize your fitness the better.

If you're concerned about brain health, remember that physical exercise is also a powerful brain booster. Physical exercise increases blood flow to the brain, which is crucial for its proper functioning. Exercise also boosts various hormones, growth factors and neuromodulators that can enhance cognitive performance and mood.

Exercise can, of course, help with improving body composition and assisting with weight loss when combined with dietary changes. A key role of exercise as we age is in supporting overall muscle mass, strength and power. After the age of 30, we start to lose between 3 and 8 per cent of muscle mass per decade. This decline seems to be particularly marked during our perimenopause and menopause years, and after the age of 60, the rate of decline increases further. Loss of muscle mass, strength and function is called sarcopenia and should be on our radar as we age.

Menopause also significantly increases bone loss and the risk of osteoporosis. Research indicates that approximately 1 in 10 women over the age of 60 are affected by osteoporosis worldwide. Resistance training and weight-bearing exercises are particularly important in supporting bone density, and by supporting muscle mass can also help prevent falls and injuries. These types of exercise also help to improve the integrity of the connective tissue and the joints, critical for injury prevention as well as for chronic conditions such as osteoarthritis.

Making movement and exercise an integral part of your daily activities is as important as brushing your teeth. If exercise is not part of your daily lifestyle, now is the time to make a change. It is not, however, a quick fix. If you're looking to change your body composition, remember, it will take time – possibly months at the very least – to see significant changes. The key is to include a variety of activities that you find enjoyable and that are sustainable for long-term results.

MOVE MORE

You don't have to be a gym goer to include more movement and exercise. Simply moving more through the day is a great place to start. However, when it comes to improving health as you age, ideally you should be looking to improve cardiorespiratory fitness, muscle mass, strength and stability. This means including a range of different activities throughout the week.

The UK government recommends at least 150 minutes of moderate-intensity (aerobic) activity such as walking or cycling, 75 minutes of vigorous activity (e.g., running), or a mixture of both spread evenly over four to five days a week, or every day. In addition, include at least two days a week of activity that strengthen muscles. If your priority is improving fitness, strength and body composition, you will need to dedicate more time and attention to activities beyond the minimum recommendations, including additional strength training, higher-intensity cardio and/or progressive exercise to meet your specific goals.

CARDIO EXERCISE

Cardio activities can vary in their intensity and duration. Walking is a great place to start, but you could also include other activities such as cycling, cross-training, rowing, dancing, running or swimming. Some of these activities will be higher impact than others. If you are struggling with joint pain or injuries, seek expert support to find the most appropriate forms of exercise. If you are looking to improve overall fitness and lose weight, you will benefit from increasing your overall activity. Why not aim for at least 60 minutes five times a week of steady-state cardio exercise. Steady-state cardio is simply a cardio workout that is a continuous, steady effort, and normally you are able to hold a conversation while exercising (walking, running, cycling, cross-trainer, etc.).

Depending on your fitness and health, you may wish to incorporate cardio exercise at a higher intensity. As we age, our cardiorespiratory capacity declines, and our lung capacity and our VO2 max drop. Having a good level of cardiorespiratory fitness enables your body to utilize oxygen more efficiently.

This is not only important for cardiovascular health and longevity, but when you are more aerobically fit, you will have more energy to enjoy doing the daily activities you like doing. This means that once or twice a week you may wish to increase the pace of your walks, cycles or runs. You could include some high-intensity interval training (HIIT).[2] HIIT is a way of training that combines quick, short, intense bursts of exercise where you are working as hard as you can with short periods of recovery. While this type of exercise may not be suitable for everyone, you certainly want to be including activities that get a sweat on and raise your heart rate. Remember, the key is to get moving more daily, so find something enjoyable that you can stick with.

THE IMPORTANCE OF STRENGTH AND POWER

We lose muscle strength about two to three times more quickly than we lose muscle mass.[3] We lose power (which is strength x speed) even more quickly. This decline is due to the atrophy in fast twitch/type II muscle fibres as we age.[4] To make matters worse, both oestrogen and progesterone support muscle mass and are involved in muscle protein synthesis. Oestrogen in particular is linked to muscle strength, power and recovery. With lower levels of oestrogen, you may find it requires more effort to get results and that recovery after exercise takes longer. If you are looking to lose fat and improve body composition, a well-designed strength training programme can help you maintain (or even gain) muscle while still losing fat.

Strength training is arguably one of the most important activities menopausal women can do to improve their overall health. Lifting heavy weights regularly – that is, at least two to three times (or more) a week – can help maintain and even improve muscle mass and strength, and support bone density.[5]

Your bone density peaks in your 20s and then gradually declines. Around menopause, this decline happens more quickly because oestrogen plays a key role in bone density. Strength training through the mechanical-loading signal stimulates bone formation. If you are serious about building muscle, aim for progressive overload in your training, as gradually increasing the weight, repetitions or intensity of exercises challenges the muscles, encouraging them to adapt and grow stronger over time.

There are many ways to load your muscles – body weight exercises, resistance bands, free weights, resistance machines can all be beneficial. If you are serious about building muscle and strength, then aim to include these types of exercises at least three to four times a week, progressively challenging yourself over time. Get expert help to ensure your movements are correct and safe to avoid injury.

STRETCHING AND STABILITY

Keeping flexible, preserving range of motion and maintaining balance and stability are all key aspects of fitness as we age, and may reduce the risk of injuries and falls. Yoga, Pilates and tai chi are all wonderful ways to improve balance, posture and flexibility. There is also some evidence that yoga may reduce the incidence of hot flushes and improve psychological wellbeing in menopausal women. Similarly, one study that involved an eight-week Pilates programme showed improvements in menopause symptoms, lumbar strength and flexibility.[6]

PELVIC FLOOR

There are oestrogen receptors in the vaginal muscles, pelvic floor and bladder, so it will come as no surprise that as oestrogen declines, muscles in this area weaken, and bladder problems and pain increase. Topical vaginal oestrogen can be helpful, especially combined with pelvic floor muscle training. If you are struggling with a pelvic health problem, speak to your GP and ask to be referred to a specialist.

GETTING STARTED

The emphasis you place on each of these different forms of exercise will, in part, be determined by your current health, fitness level and, of course, your overall health goals. If you are unsure where to begin, simply start increasing your daily steps and seek support from a qualified trainer to integrate some strength training sessions throughout the week. Ideally try to include at least 30–60 minutes of steady-state exercise daily (e.g., walking), and build in strength training several times a week.

The role of creatine during menopause

Creatine, a compound naturally found in muscle cells, plays an important role in producing energy during high-intensity exercise or muscle contraction. Creatine can be synthesized in the liver, kidneys and pancreas using three key amino acids – arginine, glycine and methionine – and obtained via the diet from animal foods (particularly red meat, fish and seafood). For those following a vegetarian or vegan diet, levels of creatine in the body may be lower, meaning supplementation may be particularly beneficial. In addition, the body's ability to produce and utilize creatine appears to decline during menopause due to the reduction in oestrogen. While creatine is often associated with exercise performance, there are numerous reasons why supplementation could be beneficial for women, particularly around menopause.[7]

- *Support muscle mass:* Creatine can be helpful in supporting and building muscle by enhancing muscle energy production, reducing fatigue when combined with resistance exercise.

- *Improved bone health:* Some research is suggesting that creatine can be helpful for bone health, particularly when combined with resistance training. Studies suggest that one of the ways it can help is via positively improving the activity of osteoblasts, the bone-forming cells, helping to promote bone formation. It may also reduce inflammation.[8] Research has shown that creatine supplementation,[9] when combined with resistance training, supports bone density in postmenopausal women.

- *Cognitive health:* Creatine supports energy production in the brain, which can enhance mental clarity, memory and cognitive function. Some studies suggest that creatine supplementation can improve short-term memory and processing speed in individuals experiencing cognitive fatigue, potentially offering a protective effect against age-related cognitive decline in women around menopause. By supporting brain energy metabolism, creatine may help improve emotional regulation and resilience during menopause. Additionally, creatine is *neuroprotective* and may help combat brain fog, which is common during menopause.

- *Energy production:* Creatine enhances ATP (adenosine triphosphate) production, which is the body's primary energy source. This boost in cellular energy can help reduce feelings of fatigue and improve overall physical and mental performance.

- *Dosage:* For general health benefits, a typical dose of creatine is around 3–5g per day. This can be taken as a supplement in powder form mixed with water or in a smoothie or protein shake. It can be taken at any time of the day.

Chapter 8

Sleep and the Circadian Rhythm

Sleep is the foundation of mental and cognitive health, vitality and overall wellbeing.

What happens during sleep can't be replicated by any state of wakefulness. Yet many women, as they approach menopause, struggle with getting quality sleep. Whether it is difficulty getting to sleep, recurrent waking, early-morning wakefulness or increased anxiety and palpitations during the night, a reduction in the quantity and quality of sleep is common. In fact, insomnia is a major complaint among perimenopausal and menopausal women – an estimated 33–51 per cent of women complain of poor sleep quality in their perimenopause and menopause years.[1] Other studies have reported an incidence of sleep disorders ranges from 16 to 47 per cent at perimenopause and 35 to 60 per cent at postmenopause.[2]

We can all recognize when we have had a bad night's sleep – it can make us feel emotional, irritable and even hungrier the following day. Even after just one bad night of sleep, there are shifts in various hormones like oestrogen, testosterone and growth hormone. Additionally, hunger hormones like ghrelin go up and leptin (involved in satiety) and insulin sensitivity go down.[3] It is no wonder we get cravings after sleep disruptions. Longer-term poor sleep can have a profound effect on our overall health. It can impact immune function, increasing the risk of infections, impair memory, mood and cognition, alter sex drive, contribute to digestive issues and hormone imbalances, and even increase our risk of heart disease. The good news is that with dietary, behavioural and lifestyle changes you can improve sleep quality for the long term.

WHY DOES OUR SLEEP CHANGE?

During perimenopause years, fluctuations and gradual declines in sex hormones have been correlated with a reduction in sleep quality.[4] Progesterone, for example, has a calming effect on the brain due to its impact on levels of the calming neurotransmitter GABA. Promoting GABA helps calm the mind, enabling us to fall asleep more readily.

Oestrogen has an effect on our circadian rhythm and temperature regulation. Since the initiation of sleep requires the body to drop its temperature by around 1–3 degrees and stay low during the night, any dysregulation of temperature (including night sweats) can result in disturbed sleep.

Women may often notice a shift in the timing of their sleep.[5] Every organ, system and cell in the body functions according to a 24-hour rhythm, which we call the circadian rhythm. Maintaining this circadian rhythm is essential to long-term health. While it is true that simply getting older can shift the circadian rhythm, one of the biggest influences for women is the decline in oestrogen.

The driver of the circadian rhythm is a part of the brain called the suprachiasmatic nucleus (SCN), which is located in the hypothalamus. The SCN is like the conductor that orchestrates circadian biological rhythms,[6] such as the rhythms of hormones, body temperature, sleep and mood. It senses light and dark and communicates to the peripheral clocks throughout the body to keep rhythm. There are oestrogen receptors in the SCN, which is one of the reasons why, when oestrogen declines, biological rhythms can get out of sync, and that, in turn, impacts sleep quality.

To make matters worse, melatonin, a key hormone involved in regulating the sleep–wake cycle (circadian rhythm), also changes during perimenopause and menopause years.[7] Melatonin is produced by the pineal gland in the brain in response to the light/dark cycle. Melatonin levels typically increase in the evening as darkness sets in, promoting sleep, and decrease in the morning as light increases, promoting wakefulness. During menopause years, women often experience earlier timing of both their body temperature rhythms and melatonin production rhythms. This combination can alter sleep patterns, making some feel sleepier earlier in the evening. It may also explain why some women wake up earlier in the morning and/or during the night and then struggle to fall back asleep.

Of course, there can be other reasons why sleep patterns may change. Health conditions such as increased stress, anxiety, depression, arthritis or back pain can all impact sleep quality. To understand how to improve sleep, it is important to highlight some of the key changes that happen to induce sleep as well as the stages of sleep.

WHY WE FEEL SLEEPY

Temperature has a profound effect on ability to fall asleep. In fact, it is the combination of a low core temperature in the circadian cycle coupled with high levels of the hormone adenosine that increases the feeling of sleepiness. Levels of adenosine build up through the day – the longer we are awake, the higher the levels of adenosine.

One of the reasons why people resort to caffeine to keep them awake is that caffeine blocks the adenosine receptors in the brain. As the effects of caffeine wear off, adenosine (which is gradually building up in the body) is suddenly able to attach to the receptors, making people feel drowsy. This is often why people experience a slump in energy and wakefulness post caffeine.

SLEEP STAGES

There are two distinct phases of sleep: non-rapid eye movement (non-REM) and rapid eye movement (REM). We cycle through these stages every 90–110 minutes on average, meaning that during an average night of sleep there will be four to five sleep cycles. Each stage of sleep is important, playing unique restoration functions including muscle recovery, hormone regulation and memory consolidation.

Within non-REM sleep, there are three stages, each progressively deeper than the last. NREM sleep is characterized by slower brain waves, reduced heart rate and relaxed muscles. It is during NREM sleep that our body repairs tissues, builds bone and muscle, and strengthens the immune system.

REM sleep is generally when we experience dreaming. In fact, our brain is very active (despite the fact we are sleeping). REM sleep is emotionally restorative as we dream – you can view REM sleep as nature's emotional regulation and therapy. REM sleep is also important for cognitive functions such as memory consolidation, learning and emotional processing.

While we cycle through these stages every 90 to 110 minutes, the proportions in terms of how long you spend in each stage changes throughout the night. Typically, the first half of the night is dominated by more deep slow-wave (non-REM) sleep, while the later part of the night has a higher proportion of REM sleep.

CORRECTING THE CLOCK

Although there can be many factors that can disrupt sleep in menopause, correcting clocks and paying attention to a regular sleep and wake cycle can improve sleep quality. A number of brain and body cues are involved in the circadian rhythm, which can, in turn, be used to improve sleep. The key ones include:

- light/dark
- temperature
- exercise
- eating patterns.

Using light to reset our biological clock and improve sleep

As light is the primary cue for the central clock, exposure to light at the right time can help improve your circadian rhythm, and impact other body processes such as digestive function and metabolic health. Studies have shown, for example, an association between greater morning light exposure, lower body fat levels and better appetite regulation.[8]

Conversely, nighttime exposure to artificial light (e.g., electronic devices), which emits shortwave blue light, suppresses melatonin secretion, interfering with sleep and other body processes. In fact, the duration and intensity of artificial light exposure at night has been associated with metabolic dysfunction, obesity and abnormal lipid profiles. Of course, part of the issue with extended evening light and wakefulness may be the tendency for late-night eating. We know from studies that late meal timing is associated with higher total daily calorie intake and increased body mass index.

But late-night eating also disrupts the metabolism, causing shifts in the clocks of organs such as the digestive organs, pancreas and liver involved in metabolic health. Late-night eating can increase the risk of insulin resistance, because when melatonin is elevated during the biological night, insulin sensitivity is impaired.[9]

Importance of morning sunlight

Morning sunlight is one of the most effective ways to set your mind and body correctly. Additionally, morning sunlight helps regulate your circadian clock, which in turn manages other biological processes, including hunger, body temperature and sleep patterns. Viewing sunlight within the first hours of waking (as soon as you can, even if through cloud cover) increases early-day cortisol release (the ideal time for elevated cortisol) and prepares the body for sleep later that night. A morning spike in cortisol will also positively influence your immune system, metabolism, mood and ability to focus during the day.

On a sunny morning, get outside for at least 5–10 minutes – this could be combined with outdoor exercise, such as a walk. Even on overcast days, there is enough natural light to have a positive benefit, but aim to be outside for at least 15–20 minutes. If it's dark on waking, flip on as many bright indoor artificial lights as possible – and then get outside as soon as the sun is out.

Afternoon sunlight to reinforce sleep

Later in the day, try to get outside. The particular wavelengths of the sun when it is low in the sky (yellows and oranges, in contrast with blue) come through even if it's overcast. Viewing sunlight in the late afternoon or evening signals the brain's circadian clock that evening is approaching, helping to transition your body into the sleep process for that night. This afternoon sunlight serves as an important anchor point for maintaining a healthy circadian rhythm.

During the day, you can also use light to improve energy and focus. Bright light can enhance the release of neurochemicals like dopamine, adrenaline and noradrenaline, which are associated with motivation, focus and drive. If you are working, try to place your desk near a window, as the natural sunlight signals the brain to stay alert and focused.

Evening light

In the late afternoon and early evening, this is the time to reduce blue light exposure (e.g., from artificial sources/electronic devices), as it can interfere with melatonin production, which is crucial for sleep. To help prepare for sleep, turn off overhead lights and opt for lamps or softer, dimmer lighting. Additionally, keeping your cortisol levels low during this time is important, as elevated cortisol can disrupt melatonin secretion and hinder your ability to wind down. Therefore, paying attention to your sleep environment is important (see Chapter 8). Ensure your room is very dark while you sleep. Even dim light exposure can impact your sleep quality.

Using temperature

Your body needs to drop in temperature by 1–3 degrees to fall and stay asleep effectively. Body temperature increases are one reason you wake up – not great if you are experiencing hot flashes or night sweats. Thus, keep your room cool and remove blankets as needed. You can also use temperature to wake you up and aid sleep. One of the reasons why a warm bath in the evening can promote sleep is that when you get out of the bath, your temperature will quickly drop, inducing sleepiness. The same approach can be used in the morning too. Having a cold shower for a couple of minutes on waking will cause a rebound in your body's temperatures. The rise will make you feel more alert.

Exercise

One of the most challenging parts of getting your body to settle down for sleep is turning off your thoughts. It's hard to get any rest at all if your mind is racing about work and a million other stressors in your life.

Regular exercise can be helpful for sleep. However, timing of exercise is important. If you are struggling to wind down at night, try to schedule exercise in the morning rather than later in the day. Exercise naturally raises cortisol levels, the hormone that helps you stay alert, and too much cortisol in the evening can interfere with melatonin production, making it harder to fall asleep. Additionally, physical activity raises your body temperature, which can increase alertness, further hindering your ability to relax as bedtime approaches.

Conversely, certain types of exercise such as meditative practices or certain forms of yoga can be used in the evening to calm the mind. Guided meditation scripts (like yoga nidra) that aim to turn off your thoughts will aid relaxation. Similarly, practising mindful breathing or breathing exercises can be helpful. These types of breathwork help because they focus the attention more on the outbreath, which initiates the parasympathetic nervous system associated with calming the mind and body.

To do this type of breathing, take a long inhale through your nose until almost to capacity. Take one more quick inhale to get a little extra air into the lungs, and then breathe out through your mouth with a long, slow exhale. This offloads the CO_2 and slows the heart rate down. Other approaches include modified box breathing, where you take a breath in (through the nose) for a count of 3, hold for 3, and then breathe out through your nose for longer – a count of 4–5. Hold for a count of 3, and then repeat.

Eating patterns

Circadian rhythms are also influenced by eating and fasting patterns. The metabolism functions differently based on the time of day. During the daytime, the body is more efficient at metabolizing and storing nutrients, while at night (when we are also fasting) the body focuses on rest, repair and lower metabolic activity. Blood glucose regulation and insulin secretion is strongly influenced by circadian rhythms. Insulin is secreted by the pancreas in the presence of glucose in the blood after eating. It aids the utilization of glucose by cells for energy and acts as an anabolic hormone, storing any excess fuel as body fat. The body appears to be more sensitive to insulin during the day, which means if you are regularly eating late at night, this may result in higher circulating insulin levels, exacerbating the problem of insulin resistance.

When and what you eat can help reset your circadian rhythm and in turn improve sleep. Your secondary timekeeper is your gut microbiome, which can help set clocks throughout the body based on periods of eating and fasting. Eating triggers the daytime circadian rhythms while fasting correlates with nighttime. This is why sticking to a regular eating pattern during the day can be beneficial. Avoid late-night eating (2–3 hours before bedtime), which can stress the digestive system, disrupt sleep and raise insulin at a time when insulin sensitivity is reduced. You may also find that eating earlier means you naturally reduce your overall calorie intake, which, in turn, can help with weight loss.

Of course, what you eat in the evening may also impact sleep. If you struggle with digestive issues or reflux, avoid fatty foods or fried foods, and keep the meal relatively light with sufficient protein and fibre to balance blood sugars. Certain foods like kiwifruit and Montmorency cherry or tart cherry juice appear to improve sleep through the impact on GABA and melatonin. In fact, eating kiwifruit with the skin on seems to decrease the amount of time to fall asleep and increases sleep duration. Drinking tart cherry juice can reduce time awake throughout the night and increase overall quantity of sleep. Chamomile tea may help you wind down in the evening due to its sedative effects.

Similarly, including foods in the evening rich in L-tryptophan may be beneficial.[10] L-tryptophan is the amino acid required for the production of serotonin (a feel good and calming neurotransmitter), and in turn the production of melatonin. Examples include dairy products, oats, poultry, fish, seeds, soy products and eggs. Combining L-tryptophan-rich foods with some carbohydrates improves its utilization by the brain.

The production of melatonin also requires certain vitamins and minerals including B vitamins (especially folate and B6), magnesium and zinc. There is also evidence that insufficient omega-3 fatty acids or an imbalance between omega-3 and omega-6 fatty acids can impact melatonin secretion (see Table 8.1).

Be mindful of the impact of caffeine on sleep patterns. Caffeine is a psychoactive stimulant that increases dopamine (making us feel alert) and blocks adenosine (which makes us sleepier). The dose and timing of coffee is what makes it helpful or harmful. Even if you don't feel the effects of late caffeine intake on sleep, cycles will likely be disrupted – particularly deep sleep. We all process caffeine at different rates, but on average the half-life of caffeine is 5–6 hours. Ideally, stop caffeine intake around 8–10 hours before the time you would like to sleep. For many people, this is likely to be around lunchtime.

Alcohol will also impact sleep quality. While alcohol is a sedative, it is not a sleep aid. Even if you find alcohol makes you sleepy, it does disrupt sleep cycles. Alcohol typically fragments sleep, so you will wake up many times throughout the night and will not have continuous sleep. Alcohol is also a potent REM sleep blocker – even one glass of wine will reduce REM sleep time. If you are struggling with sleep, avoid alcohol.

If stress is impacting your sleep, then take steps to reduce it (see Chapter 9). Cognitive behavioural therapy (CBT) has been shown to be helpful for insomnia. Acupuncture has also been found to be beneficial.[11]

Table 8.1. Key nutrients to support melatonin production

Nutrient	Food sources
Vitamin B6	Chickpeas, chicken, turkey, tuna, salmon, potato, banana, wholegrains, fortified cereals, cottage cheese, cooked spinach
Folate	Spinach, green peas, beans and pulses, avocado, rice, broccoli, asparagus, Brussels sprouts, romaine lettuce
Magnesium	Nuts and seeds, peanut butter, milk, soy milk, edamame beans, potato with skin, rice, yogurt, oats, black beans, kidney beans, salmon, halibut
Zinc	Beef, shellfish, fish, turkey, beans and pulses, sardines, dairy, eggs, rice, pumpkin seeds, oats, salmon
Omega-3 fatty acids	Fish and other seafood (especially cold-water fatty fish, such as salmon, mackerel, herring, and sardines), nuts and seeds (such as flaxseed, chia seeds and walnuts), fortified foods (e.g., eggs, juices)
L-tryptophan	Turkey, chicken, dairy, nuts, seeds, soy products (tofu, soybeans), oats, fish (salmon, tuna, cod), eggs
Vitamin D	Fatty fish, fortified foods, egg yolks, beef liver
Carbohydrates (complex)	Whole grains, whole fruits, vegetables

SUPPLEMENTS TO CONSIDER

If you have tried lifestyle and behavioural changes and are still struggling with sleep, you may wish to look at nutritional supplements to help. Always check for any interactions with medications, and seek support from your healthcare practitioner. Best taken 30–60 minutes before bed.

- 100–200mg magnesium bisglycinate or threonate
- 100–400mg L-theanine
- 1–3g glycine
- 500mg–900mg myo-inositol
- 50–100mg 5-HTP (do not take if you are taking anti-depressant SSRIs (selective serotonin reuptake inhibitors))
- 300–600mg Ashwagandha (standardized extract)
- 20–100mg CBD – start with a low dose and build up if needed (this may be useful if you are suffering with anxiety)
- 100mg apigenin (extract from chamomile).

Top tips for sleep

- Follow a regular sleep schedule. Wake up at the same time each day and go to sleep when you first start to feel sleepy. Pushing through the sleepy late-evening feeling and going to sleep too late is one reason people wake at 3am and can't fall back asleep.

- Hydrate well earlier in the day and reduce fluid intake as the day goes on. This can help prevent waking up to urinate during the night.

- Sip, don't gulp, your final beverage of the day. The speed at which you ingest fluid can affect your need to urinate. Sipping your final drink can help avoid triggering an urgent need to urinate.

- Get out early for morning light exposure. This can improve your ability to fall and stay asleep at night.

- Avoid caffeine within 8–10 hours of bedtime. The half-life of caffeine is around 5–6 hours, so stop drinking caffeine around lunchtime.

- Avoid bright lights in the evening and during the night. If you have to wake in the night to use the bathroom, try to keep light exposure to a minimum.

- Limit daytime naps to less than 30 minutes, or don't nap at all.

- If you wake up in the middle of the night but you can't fall back asleep, consider doing a meditative sleep protocol such as non-sleep deep rest or yoga nidra (you can find free guided protocols on YouTube).

- Keep the room you sleep in cool and dark. Your body needs to drop in temperature by 1–3 degrees to fall and stay asleep effectively. Body temperature increases are one reason you wake up. Thus, keep your room cool and remove blankets as needed.

- Have a warm bath about an hour before bed. Getting out of a warm bath and then allowing your temperature to drop can help you feel sleepy. Use of Epsom salts (magnesium salts) may be an additional way to calm the body and mind before bed.

- Drinking alcohol messes up your sleep. Avoid.

- Exercise earlier in the day. Exercise during the day can be a great way to improve sleep, but avoid exercising late at night as this will spike cortisol and interfere with melatonin production.

- Eat your evening meal early and avoid nighttime snacking.

- Avoid nicotine. Nicotine is a stimulant that can impact sleep.

- Include a moderate amount of starch in your evening meal. This can help you fall asleep more quickly by boosting levels of serotonin and tryptophan. Serotonin is a neurotransmitter that plays a key role in mood regulation and sleep quality, while tryptophan, an essential amino acid, is a precursor to both serotonin and melatonin, which helps regulate sleep.

- Avoid eating too much fat or protein before bed, which may affect sleep quality due to slower gastric clearance time.

- Try a warm glass of Montmorency cherry juice in the evening. This is a source of melatonin and tryptophan, and may improve sleep quality.[12]

Chapter 9

Managing Stress

Stress is inevitable. We can't control the external world but we can do our best to control how we respond to things. The perimenopause and menopause years are often a stage in a woman's life full of juggling and managing multiple commitments. This often means that stress levels are high at the same time sex hormones, which help to buffer the effects of stress, start to decline.

When you experience a short burst of stress (whether physical and psychological), there is a release of hormones such as adrenaline and cortisol from your adrenal glands, to prime the body for survival. At the same time, non-essential functions such as digestion will be suppressed. Once the threat or stressor has passed, levels of cortisol and adrenaline should return to baseline. However, when you are under chronic stress, this can impact levels of cortisol, and with it lead to negative effects on your health. For example, studies have demonstrated chronic stress results in long-term changes in the brain. There is a weakened connection between the hippocampus and prefrontal cortex, affecting motivation, focus and attention.[1] Stress can also increase amygdaloid hyper-responsivity, which leads to anxiety, and impact areas in the brain involved with learning and memory. Stress can also impact quality and quantity of sleep.

As cortisol can impact blood glucose levels, stress can contribute to blood sugar imbalances, increasing the risk of insulin resistance as well as changes in hunger and satiety, which can impact appetite. Increased levels of cortisol have been associated with increased appetite and the mobilization of fat to the central region, so stress can be a factor in the accumulation of belly fat.[2] Accumulation of visceral fat is also a well-known precursor to diabetes and cardiovascular disease. To make matters worse, as cortisol suppresses non-essential functions, such as digestion, digestive complaints such as IBS, reflux and heartburn become more common.

CHRONIC STRESS AND MENOPAUSE

During perimenopause and menopause, the adrenal glands become a bigger player in supporting levels of the sex hormones testosterone, progesterone and oestrogen, as the output from the ovaries declines. However, the adrenal glands are not as efficient at producing sex hormones when they're constantly pumping out cortisol. The more stress you experience, the more this will be compromised.

In addition, fluctuating oestrogen levels during perimenopause can act as a stressor for the body, which, in turn, may affect cortisol levels. Similarly, progesterone and dehydroepiandrosterone (DHEA) help balance the effects of cortisol, so as their levels decline, women have less of a 'stress buffer'. Chronic stress can also exacerbate the severity of various menopause symptoms, including hot flashes,[3,4,5] mood changes, sleep disturbances and changes in energy levels.

The complex relationship between cortisol, oestrogen, progesterone, testosterone and other hormones in women means that when one hormone falls out of balance, others fall too.[6] It is an intricate domino effect, and it means women entering menopause aren't just feeling psychologically stressed; they're also physically stressed. That is why it is critical to balance cortisol levels and improve resilience to stress, especially during perimenopause and menopause.

Tips for managing stress

- Exercise daily, ideally in the morning. Essential for long-term health, muscle mass and bone health, exercise can also be a great stress reliever. Try to avoid exercising late in the day, as it can elevate cortisol levels, which may interfere with melatonin production and disrupt sleep.

- Incorporate more protein into your meals – this can help to balance glucose levels, improve satiety and support muscle mass. Aim for 20–30g protein at each meal.

- Consider speaking to a qualified practitioner regarding whether bioidentical HRT could be beneficial for you.

- Make sleep a priority – improving your sleep quality can help you cope with daily stressors more effectively.

- Limit or avoid alcohol.

- Be mindful of the impact caffeine has on your levels of anxiety and stress. Switch to decaffeinated drinks if needed.

- Take time for yourself every day, even if it's just 15 to 30 minutes.

- Practise a relaxation technique, such as meditation, daily.

- Nurture positive relationships with friends and family. Social connection (e.g., your significant other, platonic friends, pets) mitigates long-term stress by releasing serotonin and suppressing tachykinin (peptides within the central and peripheral nervous system linked to symptoms such as irritability, paranoia, fear and loneliness).

- Use breathing techniques. How you breathe can impact how alert or relaxed you feel. When you inhale, the diaphragm moves down and the heart gets larger, so blood moves slower. This sends a signal to the brain to speed up the heart rate. However, when you exhale, the diaphragm moves up, the heart gets smaller and more compact, so blood moves more quickly, slowing the heart rate. One of the fastest methods to calm down when feeling stressed is to focus on longer exhales and/or practise box breathing. Other breathing techniques like Conscious Connected Breathing have been shown to help reduce stress and anxiety.[7]

- Watch your sugar intake. A diet high in sugar and refined carbo-hydrates can trigger a stress response in the body, leading to an increase in cortisol production. Instead, focus on a diet that helps keep your blood sugar levels stable. The menopause plan and recipes are designed to help balance blood glucose levels throughout the day.

SUPPLEMENTS TO CONSIDER

Various vitamins and minerals are required to support an appropriate stress response, including vitamin D, B vitamins, vitamin C, magnesium, zinc and iron. Although the nutrient quality of your diet is important during periods of stress, there are also a number of nutritional supplements that may be beneficial, including: L-theanine, lemon balm,[8] ashwagandha, CBD,[9] magnesium glycinate, rhodiola rosea, chamomile[10] and omega-3 fatty acids. Seek guidance from a qualified healthcare practitioner before starting any new supplements, to determine what is appropriate for your individual needs and health concerns.

PART 4

HOW TO EAT: THE MENOPAUSE PLAN

There is no one diet that works best for every person. The foods we consume affect numerous enzymes, metabolic processes and pathways in our body, which are influenced by our genes, our metabolism and microbiome. This means we all respond differently. In addition, our food preferences, lifestyle habits such as exercise, sleep and social interaction, and resilience to stress have a profound effect on our health. It is therefore important to personalize the diet according to your own health goals, lifestyle factors and dietary preferences.

Research is clear, however, that levels of hormones (particularly oestrogen) support key body systems and functions. This means that as you transition through the perimenopause and menopause years, you should look to address any underlying imbalances and optimize health particularly in the following areas:

- Metabolic health: Increased risk of insulin resistance, poor mitochondria function, weight gain and muscle loss.
- Cardiovascular health: Higher risk of heart disease, hypertension and inflammation.
- Immune and inflammatory balance: A shift toward chronic inflammation. Gut microbiome changes.
- Cognition and mood: Linked to memory loss, mood swings and brain fog.

The recipes and the example meal plans provided in this book aim to reset your body, address these key changes and nourish the body for long term health.

Chapter 10

Personalizing the Diet

There are two key stages of the menopause plan – Reset and Renew. If you are struggling with excess weight gain, tummy fat, blood sugar fluctuations and low energy, then the Reset meal plans can be helpful. The Reset recipes and example meal plans are designed to help you improve overall body composition, lose fat and improve metabolic health. The recipes are lower in overall carbohydrates, with a focus on protein, non-starchy vegetables, fibre and healthy fats.

The Renew stage is designed to include a wide range of nutrients and wholefoods to optimize long-term health and support key body systems like heart, brain and bone health. There is a greater emphasis on incorporating foods to modulate inflammation, support the gut microbiome and hormone health with the inclusion of phytoestrogens (see Chapter 11). All the recipes are labelled (Brain, Bone, Heart health), so you can immediately identify key recipes suited for your needs.

Regardless of whether you are starting with Reset or Renew recipes, there are some key principles to optimize your health.

CALORIES MATTER, BUT A FUNCTIONAL NUTRITION APPROACH IS KEY

The number of calories you consume each day plays a key role in weight management, but it's not the only factor to consider when it comes to health, especially during menopause. Metabolic shifts that occur during this phase – such as decreased metabolic rate and changes in how the body processes fat and carbohydrates – can make weight loss more challenging.

Inflammation, which can increase due to hormonal changes, also affects metabolism and fat storage.[1]

In addition to reducing overall calorie intake and limiting refined carbohydrates, it's important to consider the impact of these metabolic changes and address the root causes. Hormonal fluctuations, especially the decrease in oestrogen, can lead to increased fat storage, particularly around the abdominal area. Focusing on anti-inflammatory foods, such as omega-3 fatty acids, fibre-rich vegetables, and antioxidants, can be helpful in addressing inflammation and improving metabolic health.

Managing blood sugar levels by choosing whole foods, reducing stress, and incorporating regular physical activity tailored to your needs (including strength training) are also crucial. By shifting focus from just calories to a functional approach that considers hormonal balance, inflammation, the gut microbiome and metabolic health, weight loss can become more sustainable and effective during menopause.

The Reset meal plans are designed to be lower in calories while maintaining sufficient protein to support muscle mass. They also provide a good source of fibre to support metabolic health and satiety. However, it's important to remember that estimating calorie needs for weight loss is an imperfect science. It's important you do not over-restrict your calories to lose weight – your diet needs to be sustainable in the long term and rich in nutrients to support health. The Reset meal plan offers a helpful starting point, but you may need to adjust portion sizes to align with your specific weight loss and health goals.

The quality of your diet plays a vital role in long-term health, and may help alleviate some of the symptoms commonly associated with menopause. During perimenopause and menopause, it is important that nutrient intakes supports your changing health status. As an example, this is a crucial time to ensure sufficient nutrients for bone and joint health as well as omega-3 fatty acids, phospholipids and B vitamins for cognitive function and heart health. As the gut microbiome changes and your body becomes less efficient at absorbing nutrients, you need to ensure that your diet is meeting all your nutritional needs and/or supplement as needed. This is why the emphasis is on whole, nutrient-dense foods. This does not mean you have to spend hours in the kitchen – the recipes in this book are simple to make, and many can be prepared in batches for ease.

IMPORTANCE OF PROTEIN

The menopause plan emphasizes adequate protein intake, which is crucial for maintaining muscle mass, healthy body composition and overall health during this transition. As we age, the role of protein for maintaining muscle mass becomes particularly important. Protein and amino acids (which make up protein) are the essential building blocks of life. Sufficient protein is vital for maintaining and improving muscle mass and bone health.[2] While our body can use protein as an energy source, it is not a primary source of energy. The 20 amino acids that make up protein are our building blocks – not just for muscle and bones, but also for enzymes, many of our hormones and neurotransmitters, for maintaining healthy skin, hair and nails, and for and supporting immune function.

Protein has many other benefits. It is known to be thermogenic, meaning the body takes more calories to break down the same amount of protein compared to carbohydrates and fats. This may have a benefit for those looking to lose weight. Another benefit is its ability to reduce hunger and increase satiety. As anyone following a weight-loss plan knows, hunger and cravings can limit adherence to the plan. Protein helps reduce hunger via several mechanisms, including changes to hunger and satiety hormones such as ghrelin, and glucagon-like peptide-1 (GLP-1), peptide YY and cholecystokinin. Protein helps to regulate blood glucose levels, avoiding energy highs and lows throughout the day, which can often leave us feeling fatigued or craving more food. Fluctuations in blood glucose may also exacerbate menopause symptoms such as hot flashes.

One of the more overlooked benefits of including more high-protein foods in the diet is that these foods are incredibly nutritious. They tend to have a lower energy density and contain healthy fats (e.g., omega-3 fatty acids in oily fish, phospholipids in eggs) and a wealth of micronutrients.

QUALITY MATTERS

Of the 20 amino acids, there are nine essential amino acids that we must get from food as they cannot be produced by our body. This is another reason why the quality of the food we eat matters. Animal-based foods (e.g., meat, fish, eggs, poultry, dairy) contain all these essential amino acids, which is why they are sometimes referred to as complete proteins.

Plant proteins have lower digestibility and most either lack some essential amino acids or have an overall lower essential amino acid content (especially the essential amino acids methionine, lysine, leucine and tryptophan). Different plant foods contain varying amount of these amino acids. Grains, for example, are typically low in lysine but high in methionine, while beans and pulses are low in methionine and high in lysine. This means that if you are vegan, eating a variety of plant proteins daily (wholegrains, nuts, seeds, beans and pulses) can help to provide the right amount of essential amino acids. Some plant foods that have a more balanced amino acid profile include soy products (e.g., tofu, tempeh, edamame), quinoa, amaranth, buckwheat, hemp seeds, chia seeds and nutritional yeast flakes.

Leucine, isoleucine and valine, the branched-chain amino acids (BCAAs), make up about a third of muscle protein. Leucine in particular stimulates protein synthesis in muscle, and therefore becomes particularly important in maintaining muscle as we age.[3,4] Useful dietary sources of leucine include meat, fish, dairy, soy and nuts.

HOW MUCH PROTEIN?

How much protein we need depends on our age, body weight, lean muscle mass and activity levels. There is evidence that as we get older, we require more protein for the same effect due to anabolic resistance. That is, it is more difficult for our bodies to utilize protein for maintaining or gaining muscle mass. Ensuring adequate protein intake stimulates muscle protein synthesis (MPS) to achieve a positive protein balance, which, in turn, and with the right exercise, leads to more muscle over time.

As we age, the general recommendations for protein is an intake of around 1–1.2g/kg body weight per day. For a 9-stone (57kg) woman, this would equate to 57–68g protein per day. However, this level of protein intake may not be sufficient, especially for women going through the menopause transition, a time marked by hormonal shifts that can accelerate muscle loss and increase fat accumulation. To support muscle maintenance and growth, promote fat loss and improve overall body composition during this stage, research suggests that daily protein intake should be significantly higher, between 1.4 and 2.0g protein per kilogram of body weight.[5] So, for a 9-stone woman, this may be 80–114g per day. In order to achieve this, the 9-stone woman should aim for at least a quarter of her plate to be lean, protein-rich foods. Although the Reset meal plans contain over 100g protein on average daily, some women may actually need a higher intake than this.

Remember that protein is essential for supporting muscle mass and healthy bones, but you also need to combine this with the appropriate amount of the right type of exercise. Resistance training combined with adequate protein intake is necessary to maximize muscle growth and strength and support bone health as we age. While the total daily amount of protein is most important when it comes to maintaining or improving muscle mass, how you spread your protein out through the day can also be beneficial. Studies indicate that spreading protein intake evenly across the day rather than in just one meal appears more effective in stimulating muscle protein synthesis.

As a general guide, around 0.25–0.4g/kg body weight per meal is recommended, or around 20g–40g protein per meal.[6,7]

SLOW, NOT NO, CARBOHYDRATES

This is not a very low-carbohydrate diet, but it does reduce overall carbohydrates while focusing on complex carbohydrates to improve overall metabolic health. Since the risk of insulin resistance increases around menopause, it is important to be mindful of the type and amount of carbohydrates consumed. There is a greater emphasis on whole plant foods (wholegrains, vegetables, fruits, legumes, nuts, seeds), which provide not only carbohydrates but also plenty of fibre, vitamins, minerals and antioxidants.

Carbohydrates are often classed as 'simple' or 'complex'. Simple carbohydrates (sugars) are found in refined foods such as processed foods, cookies, breakfast cereals, white bread, etc. These are broken down readily in the body, resulting in rapid blood sugar spikes that often lead to fluctuating blood sugar levels throughout the day, affecting energy levels, mood and appetite. They are also very low in essential vitamins, minerals and fibre. Many processed carbohydrate foods (think cakes, cookies and pastries) will also contain added fats and calories.

Complex carbohydrates (found in wholegrains, legumes, whole fruit, vegetables, nuts and seeds) tend to be naturally high in vitamins, minerals and antioxidants, and are an important source of fibre. As such, they take longer to digest than refined carbohydrates, meaning a more gradual rise in blood glucose after eating. This helps maintain more even energy throughout the day, reducing dramatic spikes in insulin.

It is not just the quality of carbohydrates eaten that impacts blood glucose spikes but also the quantity consumed. You will experience more balanced blood glucose levels through the day by watching your carbohydrate portions and combining carbohydrates with proteins and healthy fats at both mealtimes and as snacks. As women around menopause have a tendency to become more insulin resistant, reducing their intake of refined carbohydrates and focusing on the quality and quantity of carbohydrates eaten becomes particularly important.

How much total carbohydrates you should eat in a day will be influenced by various factors, including overall calorie requirements, activity levels and health goals and concerns. If you are concerned about insulin resistance and wish to follow the Reset, a good rule of thumb is around 30–50g carbohydrates per meal.

WHOLEGRAINS

Grains are the seeds of cereal plants. Wholegrains contain the entire grain, which is made up of the fibre-rich outer layer (the bran), the nutrient-packed inner part (the germ) and the central starchy part (the endosperm). Wholegrains provide plenty of fibre and an array of other nutrients that are important for menopause, including B vitamins, essential fatty acids (omega-3 fats), protein, antioxidants including vitamin E, selenium and minerals such as copper, manganese and magnesium.

FOOD SENSITIVITIES

As we age, our digestive system undergoes a number of changes that can affect our ability to digest certain foods. Reduced production of stomach acid may lead to difficulties in breaking down certain foods. This, coupled with changes in the microbiome composition, may impact our immune response, shifting the body into a more reactive and pro-inflammatory state.[8,9] Previous foods that were tolerated may become more problematic. Symptoms such as IBS and reflux are often more noticeable around menopause.[10]

In addition, wholegrains like wheat, barley and rye contain gluten, which may, for some, cause digestive symptoms (like bloating, constipation and abdominal pain) and non-gastrointestinal (GI) symptoms (such as headaches, brain fog, fatigue or joint pain). While coeliac disease, which is an autoimmune disease, is well documented, affecting around 1 in 100 people, non-coeliac gluten sensitivity is less well researched but is believed to affect between 1 and 13 per cent of the population.[11,12]

Women around menopause may be more susceptible to food sensitivities due to these changes in digestive secretions, bowel motility and microbiome shifts. If you suspect gluten or other foods are causing a problem, it is important to seek medical advice before cutting out foods or food groups.

IMPORTANCE OF PLANTS

Eating plant-based foods does not mean you have to be vegetarian or vegan, but a higher intake of a wide variety of plant foods will provide plenty of fibre, prebiotics, vitamins, minerals, antioxidants and healthy fats. This can, in turn, be beneficial for overall digestive health, microbiome diversity, cognitive health and cardiovascular health, and may help regulate appetite and promote healthy body composition.

EMPHASIZE GUT HEALTH

During perimenopause and menopause, a number of changes occur that impact gut health. The menopause plan includes probiotic-rich foods, fibre and prebiotics to support a healthy, diverse microbiome and overall digestive health.

NOURISHING FATS

Your brain and body need the right fats. This is why the recipes in this book focus on beneficial monounsaturated fats and omega-3 and omega-6 fats. There is also an emphasis on phospholipids such as choline-rich foods that are vital for cellular health and cognitive health.

IMPORTANCE OF FATS

Dietary fats play an important role in the diet. In addition to being a source of energy, fats are required for hormone production, cell membrane health, brain function and nutrient absorption, and are a source of valuable fat-soluble vitamins (vitamins D, A, E and K).

Dietary fat is more energy dense than protein and carbohydrates (fat contains 9 kcal/g) and so consuming too much can quickly increase overall calorie intake, but adding a little fat to a meal tends to leave you feeling more satiated, especially when combined with protein. Fat can also improve the absorption of certain plant nutrients like lycopene (found in tomatoes).

There are broadly three types of fat: saturated fatty acids, monounsaturated fatty acids and polyunsaturated fatty acids. Within polyunsaturated fatty acids, there are omega-3 and omega-6 fatty acids. The omega-3 fats include alpha-linolenic acid (ALA), eicosapentaenoic acid (EPA) and docosahexaenoic acid (DHA). ALA is mostly found in plants, while EPA and DHA are mostly found in animal foods such as fatty fish. All foods that contain fat will actually contain a variety of these of fats in different proportions.

Another type of fat called trans fats (often listed on labels as partially hydrogenated vegetable oil) is created during a process known as hydrogenation. These are found in various processed foods (like pastries, crisps, etc.) and should be avoided.

Saturated fats are mainly found in animal products and certain plant foods like coconut and palm oil. They are heat stable and useful for cooking at higher temperatures.

Omega-3 fatty acids are essential fats (meaning we need to get them from our diet), and DHA and EPA in particular have been shown to possess a range of health benefits, including supporting cognition and mood, heart health, improved joint and bone health and immune function. In fact, omega-3 fats have strong anti-inflammatory properties.

ALA[13] is mostly found in plant foods (e.g., flaxseed, chia seeds, pumpkin seeds, hemp and walnuts) and is an essential precursor of EPA or DHA. However, the conversion of ALA to EPA and DHA is poor, with as little as 4–6 per cent converted to DHA after consumption. The best food sources of DHA and EPA are oily fish (e.g., salmon, mackerel, sardines, trout, anchovies, fresh tuna).

Omega-6 fatty acids are found in a wide range of foods such as nuts, seeds, grains and vegetable oils. As these are more easily found in foods, we often have an imbalanced intake of omega-6 to omega-3. If you are looking to promote health and lower inflammation, increasing your intake of omega-3-rich foods and reducing overall omega-6 intake can be beneficial.

Monounsaturated fats are found in foods such as olive oil, avocado and various nuts and seeds. They have been shown in studies to have cardioprotective properties and anti-inflammatory effects.[14] Abundant in the Mediterranean diet, this is one of the reasons why a Mediterranean style of eating appears to have many longevity and heart-healthy benefits. Of course, it is worth mentioning that we consume many of these fats in foods, not just as oils. As such, these foods will contain many other beneficial nutrients, vitamins, minerals and antioxidants. For example, nuts are good sources of protein, fibre, B vitamins, vitamin E, magnesium, zinc, calcium, potassium and phytosterols.

For health, we want a combination of saturated, monounsaturated and polyunsaturated fats. During menopause, particular focus should be on increasing omega-3 fatty acids and monounsaturated fats to support long-term health and lower inflammation.

PHOSPHOLIPIDS

Phospholipids are unique molecules. They are major components of cell membranes and are also involved in various cellular processes. Some, like phosphatidylcholine and phosphatidylserine, have particular benefits for brain health, mood and cognition. In fact, the brain is one of the richest tissues in terms of phospholipid content. About 50 per cent of the dry weight of the brain is lipid, and almost half of that is phospholipid associated with cell membranes. Studies have shown improvements in cognitive health, resilience to stress and overall brain health with an increased intake of phospholipids.[15] This is particularly important around menopause since lower oestrogen increases the need for choline, which is required for the production of acetylcholine involved in mood and memory.[16] (A list of choline-rich foods can be found in Chapter 5).

Tackle inflammation

Menopause is really an inflammatory transition in a woman's life, marked by several physiological changes. This shift to a more inflammatory state can manifest as pain, muscle stiffness, brain fog, depression, osteoarthritis and a reduction in bone density. One of the key reasons for this increased inflammation is the decline in oestrogen levels. Oestrogen acts as both a natural anti-inflammatory agent and an antioxidant. This reduction in oestrogen exacerbates the impact of oxidative stress and damage linked to longer-term health concerns associated with menopause. The recipes therefore avoid foods that may exacerbate inflammation, such as processed foods, processed meats, sugar, caffeine and an excess of omega 6 rich foods.[17] Instead, there is a focus on foods rich in antioxidants (colourful fruits, vegetables, nuts and seeds), omega-3 fatty acids (oily fish, flaxseed and chia seeds), spices like turmeric and ginger, phytoestrogens (see Chapter 11), green tea, mushrooms and monounsaturated fats (olive oil, avocado).

Time-restricted eating

The timing of your meals can help regulate your natural body clock and improve sleep. Eating at regular times during the day and avoiding late-night eating can greatly improve energy levels, digestion and sleep.[18] For weight loss, while it may not necessarily have any advantages over simple calorie restriction, one potential benefit of time-restricted eating is that it is often easier not to over-eat. By condensing food intake into fewer hours over the day, studies show you can naturally reduce calories.[19] Studies have also demonstrated that time-restricted eating reduces fasting blood glucose and improves insulin sensitivity.[20] This does not mean you have to fast for long periods of time. Simply eating your evening meal early and going 12–14 hours overnight with no food can be beneficial.

ALCOHOL

Alcohol is actually a macronutrient. It is calorie dense (containing 7 kcal/g) and has no nutritional or health benefits. This is why alcohol is considered 'empty calories'. In fact, alcohol that is converted to acetaldehyde in the body is a known toxin, and produces substantial stress and damage to the cells. If you are trying to lose weight, be mindful that alcohol can disrupt metabolic health. The processing of alcohol that occurs via the liver delays fat oxidation. To make matters worse, many people find themselves mindlessly eating when drinking alcohol, which can further impact ability to lose fat.

Alcohol affects the female body differently than it affects the male body. This is caused by females' lower levels of dehydrogenase enzymes, the enzyme that breaks down alcohol, coupled with typically a higher fat/water ratio in the female body. This can cause alcohol levels to rise more quickly after ingestion in women than in men, which makes females more vulnerable to alcohol's harmful effects. For women transitioning through menopause, alcohol may also exacerbate symptoms such as hot flashes and night sweats.[21]

Alcohol impacts the body in other ways too. It is problematic for the gut microbiome, which is altered during menopause, as it disrupts the balance of beneficial bacteria, encouraging dysbiosis and disrupting the health of the gut lining. Alcohol can also increase risk of cancer, including breast cancer. It increases the conversion of testosterone to oestrogen via a process called aromatization, which can, in turn, contribute to hormone imbalances.

Because alcohol is water- and fat-soluble, it can also cross the blood–brain barrier, impacting brain chemistry and neural circuits. Even low to moderate drinking can impact brain health and function, neurotransmitter activity and resilience to stress.[22]

Sleep problems, which are commonly associated with menopause, are impacted by alcohol. While many people think a glass of wine might be nice to make them sleepy, it actually disrupts quality of sleep – slow-wave sleep and REM sleep, both of which are essential for getting a restorative night's sleep, are disrupted. Alcohol typically leads to multiple bouts of waking up during the night, which you may not even be aware of, and the result is less rested sleep.

In view of this, it is best to avoid or minimize your intake of alcohol, particularly if you wish to lose weight or are struggling with hot flashes.[23] Be mindful that recent research indicates that no amount of alcohol is entirely without risk.

Chapter 11

Nourishing a Healthy Gut: The Importance of Diet Diversity

Gut microbiota are the trillions of microorganisms, including bacteria, viruses and fungi, that live in the digestive tract. Not only are they vital for healthy digestion, but research is showing us that they also affect pretty much all aspects of health, including the immune system, hormone balance, cognition and mood, as well as heart, skin and bone health. A diverse gut microbiota is considered a marker of resilience and overall health, and this diversity is shaped significantly by dietary patterns, among other lifestyle factors.

During perimenopause, menopause and beyond, many women notice changes in their digestive health – this may include IBS symptoms, reflux, heartburn, bloating or changes in bowel movements. Research suggests that the decline in oestrogen during menopause can influence the gut microbiome,[1] affecting both the small and large intestines, as well as the vaginal microbiome. These changes may lead to increased inflammation, mucosal damage and altered immune responses. The health of the gut microbiome is also closely linked to the vaginal microbiome, with the balance of beneficial bacteria being disrupted due to increased vaginal pH caused by reduced oestrogen. This shift in the vaginal microbiome, characterized by a decrease in *Lactobacillus* levels, has been associated with symptoms such as urinary urgency, incontinence and an increased risk of urinary tract infections. Therefore, maintaining a healthy gut and vaginal microbiome is essential for managing many menopause-related symptoms.

Reduced oestrogen levels during perimenopause and menopause can impact the health of the digestive tract, which contains a high concentration of oestrogen receptors. This hormonal shift may contribute to increased gut permeability, allowing harmful substances to cross the intestinal lining promoting inflammation.

Oestrogen decline can also influence the composition of the gut microbiota, potentially reducing the diversity and abundance of beneficial bacteria. As a result, the production of short-chain fatty acids (SCFAs), key compounds that help maintain gut barrier integrity and regulate inflammation may decrease.

This highlights the importance of consuming a fibre-rich diet to support a diverse gut microbiome. Additionally, plant foods rich in phytoestrogens can offer extra benefits. These natural compounds bind to oestrogen receptors throughout the body, including the gut, and have been shown to positively influence the diversity and balance of gut microbes.

Interestingly, gut dysbiosis can also affect hormone metabolism, making this interplay especially relevant for perimenopausal women. Including phytoestrogen-rich foods such as ground flaxseeds, sesame seeds and soy products (e.g. edamame, tofu, tempeh) can therefore support gut health and help ease symptoms related to hormonal fluctuations during menopause.

GUT HEALTH AND HORMONE HEALTH – THE ESTROBOLOME

The perimenopausal years are typically associated with fluctuating hormone levels. The health of the gut during this stage in life can significantly impact hormone regulation, and vice versa. The gut microbiome plays a key role in metabolizing and modulating various hormones, including oestrogen. As oestrogen levels decline at menopause, changes in the gut microbiome occur, potentially affecting hormone balance and worsening menopausal symptoms.

Certain microbes in the gut, collectively referred to as the estrobolome, influence how much oestrogen is available for recirculation.[2] These microbes produce an enzyme called beta-glucuronidase, which deconjugates oestrogen (and various toxins) in the gut, allowing it to be reabsorbed into the bloodstream. A well-balanced estrobolome helps regulate circulating oestrogen levels, whereas an imbalance in gut bacteria may alter beta-glucuronidase activity, contributing to oestrogen deficiencies or excesses. Emerging research has linked this microbial imbalance to menopause-related symptoms such as hot flashes, mood changes, sleep disturbances and metabolic alterations.

Additionally, oestrogen plays a role in gut barrier function, helping to maintain the integrity of the intestinal lining. As oestrogen declines during menopause, gut permeability may increase, leading to inflammation and digestive discomfort. Common menopausal concerns, including weight gain, insulin resistance and irritable bowel syndrome (IBS), may be exacerbated by these gut changes.

To support gut health during menopause, it is important to consume a diverse range of plant-based foods. Fibre-rich foods such as wholegrains, legumes and vegetables promote a more balanced microbiome, while prebiotics (found in onions, leeks, bananas and flaxseeds) help feed beneficial gut bacteria. Fermented foods such as sauerkraut, kimchi, miso, pickles, natural yoghurt and kefir introduce probiotics that further support gut health. Additionally, polyphenol-rich foods, including berries, green tea and dark chocolate, have been shown to benefit gut bacteria and overall wellbeing.

The role of fibre

Fibre is a type of complex carbohydrate found in plants. Unlike other carbohydrates, we cannot break them down during digestion, so they pass through into the large intestine, where the majority of our gut microbes live. Our gut microbes digest this fibre for us, and by doing so produce a number of beneficial compounds and metabolites including SCFAs, such as butyrate, propionate and acetate. These SCFAs nourish the gut lining but also influence many other body systems and functions including brain health, immune function and metabolism.

The current recommendation is to consume 30g of fibre daily, yet most people fail to get this amount. Even upping your fibre by an extra 8g per day has been linked to reduced risk of heart disease, type 2 diabetes and colorectal cancer.[3] Consuming sufficient fibre with adequate water through the day can also ensure regular bowel movements. Constipation often gets worse around menopause, as declining oestrogen levels impact the motility of the gut, slowing the passage of food through the intestinal tract. Adequate fibre in the diet can also have beneficial effects on cholesterol levels, prevent blood sugar spikes and keep you feeling fuller for longer.

The easiest way to increase your intake of fibre is to include more plants and a greater variety of plants in your diet. Following the results from the American Gut Project,[4] it is clear that a diverse plant-based diet is beneficial for gut health. This is one of the key aspects of the menopause plate – a diverse, colourful, plant-focused diet.

Studies have also supported this approach. A study of more than 17,000 menopausal women showed a 19 per cent reduction in hot flashes for those who ate more vegetables, fruit, fibre and soy compared to the control group.[5]

Of course, when it comes to fibre, it is important to take it slowly. If you are not used to eating a lot of fibre, you will want to gradually increase your intake over a number of weeks. There are plenty of recipes in this book that are quick and easy to make, and that are a good place to start.

PREBIOTICS

Both dietary fibre and prebiotics are beneficial to health. Prebiotics include both fibre and non-fibre compounds that serve as food for beneficial microbes in our gut. We can't digest prebiotics, but certain beneficial microbes can. Prebiotics are selectively utilized by resident beneficial microbes – this means they have targeted effects on our bacteria. Most microbes won't be affected. It is this selective utilization that distinguishes prebiotics from fibre. Prebiotics encourage the activities of microbes that have beneficial functions, including those commonly used as probiotics (*Lactobacillus* and *Bifidobacterium*). Prebiotics help modulate our immune system and satiety, and promote metabolic health (insulin health and healthy lipids). Examples of prebiotics include prebiotic fibres, resistant starches and polyphenols (a type of phytonutrient found in foods like berries and apples). Prebiotics encourage both the growth of health-promoting bacteria species as well as enhancing their activity. Indeed, the production of organic compounds by beneficial bacteria such as SCFAs (butyrate, propionate and acetate) is greatly supported by prebiotic foods.

PROBIOTICS

Probiotics are foods or supplements that contain live bacteria, which are potentially beneficial to human health. Common probiotics are certain strains of *Lactobacillius* and *Bifidobacteria*, *Saccharomyces boulardii* and *Bacillus coagulans*, but there many others. Some foods, such as fermented milk products (plain yogurt, kefir), kombucha, sauerkraut, miso, kimchi, tempeh, natto and certain pickles are naturally rich in probiotics, and may therefore help balance gut microbiota and modulate the immune response. Emerging studies suggest that fermented foods particularly kefir, can be beneficial during menopause. Research has shown that kefir improves quality of life and reduces sleep disturbances and improve mood in postmenopausal women.[6] Additionally, fermented foods like kimchi can aid in managing IBS, a common issue during menopause, and support a healthy gut microbiome.[7] While some probiotics may have a transitory effect, meaning they do not settle in the gut for life, they still may have an influence on gut health and in creating a more suitable environment for a diverse microbiome. For this reason, fermented foods are widely used throughout the menopause plan.

IMPORTANCE OF COLOUR AND VARIETY

To support a healthy microbiome, plants should be a central focus of our diet. Both quality and variety matter in order to provide us with essential nutrients, antioxidants and fibre to support health, including gut health. We want to include a wide range of colourful plants and plenty of variety daily. Each plant will provide us with a different range of nutrients and phytochemicals – there is no one magic superfood.

Phytochemicals or phytonutrients are plant compounds that have been shown to have a number of beneficial effects in our body, including supporting the immune system, improving heart and blood vessel health, supporting brain health and promoting healthy oestrogen metabolism. Studies have also shown that eating more plant foods is associated with better brain health and lower inflammation. It is these phytochemicals that give plants their colour and influence their flavour. The more colour in our diet and the greater the variety of plants, the larger the number of phytochemicals we will consume.

With some foods, the antioxidant content increases when cooked. This is particularly true for those foods rich in carotenoids, found in red, orange, yellow and green foods. Cooked tomato products, for example, result in most of the carotenoid lycopene being absorbed by the body. Lycopene is also fat-soluble, which means fat aids absorption. Therefore, an ideal combination could be making a cooked tomato sauce with a splash of olive oil. Try not to overcook vegetables – generally, lightly steaming vegetables is more likely to preserve nutrients better than boiling. Remember, too, that for many fruits and vegetables the highest levels of phytonutrients is found in the skin, so it not always necessary to peel fruit and vegetables – good news if you are short on time.

Table 11.1. Various food colours and their nutrients

Colour	Examples of phytonutrients	Menopause benefits	Food examples
Red	Anthocyanins Lycopene Quercetin Proanthocyanidins Ellagic acid Ellagitannins Fisetin	Anti-bacterial (e.g., gut, urinary) Anti-cancer Anti-inflammatory Brain health Cell protection Heart health	Apples Beans (adzuki, kidney, red) Cranberries Cherries Plums Pomegranate seeds Radishes Raspberries Red onions Red pepper Strawberries Tomatoes Watermelon

Orange	Alpha-carotene Beta-carotene Beta-cryptoxanthin Bioflavonoids Carotenoids Curcuminoids Naringenin	Anti-inflammatory (e.g., joints, bones) Blood vessel health Brain health Cell protection Heart health Eye health	Apricots Butternut squash Cantaloupe melon Carrots Mango Orange Papaya Sweet potato Turmeric root
Yellow	Lutein Rutin Zeaxanthin	Anti-inflammatory (e.g., joints) Cell protection Digestive health Eye health Heart health Immune health	Apples Bananas Corn Ginger root Jackfruit Passionfruit Pineapple Yellow pepper
Green	Catechins Chlorogenic acid Chlorophyll Epigallocatechin gallate Glucosinolates Hydroxytyrosol Indole-3-carbinol Isoflavones Isothiocyanate Oleocanthal Oleuropein Phytosterols Phenols Sulforaphane Tannins	Anti-cancer Anti-inflammatory Blood vessel health Bone health Brain health Cell protection Heart health Hormone balance Metabolic health	Asparagus Avocado Broccoli Brussels sprouts Cabbage Celery Courgettes Cucumbers Edamame/soybeans Green beans Green peas Green tea Leafy greens (e.g., lettuce, kale, watercress) Kiwifruit Pak choi
Blue/ purple	Anthocyanidins Hydroxystilbenes Procyanidins Pterostilbene Resveratrol	Anti-inflammatory Blood vessel health Bone health Brain health Cell protection Digestive health Heart health Liver health	Aubergine Berries (e.g., blueberries, blackberries) Black beans Black olives Black rice Figs Plums Prunes Raisins

cont.

Colour	Examples of phytonutrients	Menopause benefits	Food examples
White/ brown	Allicin Allyl sulfides Cellulose (fibre) Lignans Lignins Sesamin Sesamol Tannins Theobromine	Anti-cancer Anti-inflammatory Blood vessel health Bone health Brain health Cell protection Digestive health Heart health Immune health Metabolic health	Cauliflower Cocoa Coffee Dates Flaxseed Garlic Legumes (e.g., chickpeas, butterbeans) Mushrooms Nuts and seeds (including nut and seed butters) Onions Pears Tea Wholegrains (e.g., oats, brown rice, quinoa)

POLYPHENOLS

Polyphenols are an example of phytochemicals found in plant-based foods and drinks. They have antioxidant properties, making them beneficial in protecting the body from the effects of oxidative stress. This is particularly important around menopause, since oestrogen itself has antioxidant properties. Polyphenols have many health benefits such as reducing the risk of heart disease, type 2 diabetes and certain cancers. Polyphenols also support the growth of beneficial bacteria in the gut. This is because up to 95 per cent of the polyphenols we consume travel undigested to our large intestine where they are broken down by beneficial gut microbes.[8] This makes polyphenols a type of prebiotic.

Polyphenols promote the growth of beneficial bacteria like *Bifidobacterium* and *Lactobacillus*.[9] Certain polyphenols have a positive effect on another beneficial bacteria called *Akkermansia muciniphila*. This beneficial microbe accounts for up to 4 per cent of intestinal bacteria and is associated with lean body mass and obesity prevention. *Akkermansia muciniphila*, along with other beneficial bacteria, supports the health of the gut lining, sometimes called the intestinal barrier, which can become compromised around menopause. The intestinal barrier works to allow nutrients, electrolytes and water to leave the gut and travel to areas of the body that need them. And it protects us from invading pathogens, potential allergens and toxins that could adversely affect our health.

Polyphenols help regulate the composition of beneficial gut bacteria, which can positively influence brain function and mood.[10] Polyphenols may have neuroprotective effects by reducing inflammation and oxidative stress, which can influence brain health, particularly as we age. Changes in the gut microbiome during menopause and ageing may be associated with an increased risk of neurodegenerative diseases, such as Alzheimer's. By consuming polyphenol-rich foods, we support a healthy gut microbiome, which, in turn, may produce compounds that promote overall health, including potential neuroprotective effects. The easiest way to ensure our diet is rich in polyphenols is to include a variety of colourful plant foods. This is the essence of the menopause plan.

So, it is important to maintain a healthy digestive tract with a plant-focused diet rich in fibre,[11] prebiotics and probiotics.

ROLE OF PHYTOESTROGENS

Phytoestrogens are oestrogen-like compounds derived from plants, which are structurally similar to oestradiol. As such these compounds can have a mild oestrogenic effect. When our levels of oestrogens are low around the menopause, phytoestrogens in foods such as soy and flaxseed appear to bind preferentially to oestrogen receptors, particularly the beta receptors that are present in many areas of the brain, gut, skin, immune cells and endothelial cells in our cardiovascular system.[12] They may act as weak oestrogen receptor agonists or antagonists, depending on tissue type and circulating hormone levels.

Phytoestrogens have been shown to act as neuroprotectors and anti-oxidants, helping to reduce the risk of Alzheimer's disease and cognitive decline. They may also influence neuromodulators like serotonin, which help balance mood. Other studies have demonstrated the protective effects of phytoestrogens on cardiovascular disease.[13] This is likely to be due to a number of actions including reduction of total cholesterol, LDL cholesterol, increasing HDL cholesterol, lowering blood pressure, C reactive protein, triglycerides and fasting blood glucose levels. Although the data is mixed, there are also studies to suggest that consumption of isoflavones (particularly soy) may have a positive impact on hot flashes, vaginal atrophy, sleep disturbances, bone mineral density and skin health.[14] Some evidence suggests they may help reduce the frequency and severity of hot flashes, though results vary by individual and dose.

The main groups of phytoestrogens are isoflavones, stilbene, coumestan, flavonols and lignans; the most studied are isoflavones (particularly soy) and lignans (such as flaxseed).

Most of the phytoestrogens present in the diet are inactive compounds, which, on consumption, have to go through series of enzymatic changes in the gut to form the active phytoestrogenic compounds. These transformations are mediated by the gut microbiota, and not all individuals have the bacteria needed to convert isoflavones into more potent metabolites like equol. So a healthy gut is important to optimize their benefits.[15] For this reason, fermented products such as miso, natto and tempeh are likely to be particularly beneficial.

Isoflavones, one of the main groups of phytoestrogens, are found in soybeans and other legumes (e.g., chickpeas, beans and lentils) as well as fruits like pomegranate seeds. The amount of isoflavones needed for health benefits is around 40–70mg/day, or an average of 50mg/day. The average consumption of isoflavones in Asian society is 15–50mg per day, while in Western countries it is only about 2mg per day. So, to optimize the benefits, you may need to increase your intake. Research suggests that soy isoflavones may help reduce incidence of hot flashes and support bone health post menopause.[16] These effects are more consistent in populations with long-term soy intake.

The stilbene group includes resveratrol, found in grapes and peanuts. Coumestans are found in legumes and certain vegetables like broccoli, cabbage, spinach and alfalfa sprouts. The main sources of lignans are flaxseed and sesame seeds, although they are also present in other seeds and grains (like oats and rice), and fruits such as peaches and vegetables (e.g., broccoli). Flaxseeds are incredibly rich in lignans. In fact, they contain up to 800 times more lignans than other plant foods. Some studies suggest that lignans in flaxseed may help lower the risk of breast cancer in postmenopausal women, although more long-term studies are needed to confirm this effect.[17]

Flavonols include plants rich in quercetin and rutin, such as buckwheat, apples, onion and pomegranate seeds. Remember that these foods also contain a wealth of additional nutrients that are beneficial to health, including fibre, antioxidants, vitamins and minerals. By including a diverse range of these plants, you will ensure a greater intake of nutrients as well as phytoestrogens.[18]

Table 11.2. Food sources of phytoestrogens by category
(Rich or notable sources of isoflavones, lignans and other phytoestrogen compounds)

Category	Examples	Key phytoestrogen type	Comment
Soy products	Tempeh, tofu, miso, natto, edamame	Isoflavones (genistein, daidzein)	Primary dietary source
Seeds	Flaxseed, sesame seeds	Lignans	Highest lignan content
Legumes	Chickpeas, lentils, butterbeans	Isoflavones (lower levels)	Modest contributors
Sprouts	Alfalfa, broccoli sprouts	Coumestans (e.g. coumestrol)	Minor but active
Fruits	Pomegranate, red grapes, plums	Lignans, flavonoids	Low to moderate content
Vegetables	Cabbage, spinach, broccoli	Coumestans, lignans	Minor contributors
Grains	Oats, rye, barley, wheat bran	Lignans, flavonoids	Small amounts

To increase your daily intake of phytoestrogens:

- Try seeded crackers (see Tomato Flaxseed Crackers on page 225).
- Switch to linseed or seeded breads (see Buckwheat, Fruit and Seed Bread on page 222 and Cranberry Cottage Cheese Bread on page 224).
- Make your own seed and nut-based granola (see Chai Spiced Granola on page 142).
- Use a range of wholegrains like quinoa or buckwheat in salads

or porridge (see, for example, Slow-Roasted Lamb with Citrus Quinoa Salad on page 180).

- Toss nuts and seeds or sprouted beans in salads.
- Make up trail mixes with dried fruits, nuts and seeds.
- Snack on cooked edamame beans or roasted chickpeas/lentils (see Salt and Vinegar Roasted Chickpeas on page 226).
- Blend silken tofu into soups or desserts (see, for example, Roasted Broccoli and Fennel Soup on page 161 and Matcha Green Tea Mint Ice Cream on page 231).
- Blend butterbeans or cannellini beans into soups for a creamy texture.

Chapter 12

Reset and Renew

GETTING STARTED – THE RESET STAGE

The Reset stage of the menopause plan focuses on improving your body composition. Whether you have a few kilograms to lose or more, or you've started to notice more belly fat, these recipes and example meal plans can help. While the principles outlined in Chapters 10 and 11 apply throughout the recipes, you will notice that the Reset recipes are typically higher in protein and lower in carbohydrates.

Reset recipes for breakfast, lunch or dinner contain a minimum of 20g protein per serving. You'll also notice certain snacks and desserts labelled as Reset. These options are typically lower in calories and are moderate to low in carbohydrates. The recipes are also lower in carbohydrates, with less than 45g per meal. However, remember this is a guide only. To support a healthy weight loss and improve body composition, pay attention to overall calories and protein intake. Some people will require a little more protein based on their size and activity levels. As a general guide in the example meal plans, contain a minimum of 100g protein – the macronutrient split is around 30–35 per cent carbohydrates, protein 30–35 per cent, fats 30–40 per cent. Note this is a guide only – you may need to tweak your calorie intake based on your weight-loss goals.

Building your Reset plate

Aim for three meals a day, with an optional snack. Try to spread your meals out through the day, and avoid grazing/snacking.

Plan your meals around protein and vegetables. Start with *protein*, which should make up about a quarter of your plate. Protein is essential for maintaining muscle during weight loss, and keeps you feeling full for longer, so be sure to prioritize it in every meal.

Next, fill your plate (at least half) with fibrous, low-starchy vegetables (e.g., leafy greens, green beans, courgettes, asparagus, kale, broccoli, spinach, cauliflower, pak choi, Brussels sprouts, cabbage, sauerkraut, kimchi, aubergine, salad greens, cucumber, mushrooms). You may also wish to include one or two pieces of fruit daily.

Fats are crucial for health, satiety and proper hormone function. Include healthy fat sources like avocado, olive oil, nuts and seeds. These are generally included in the recipes, either as a dressing, an addition to the dish or for cooking with.

Include some dairy (or fortified dairy alternatives) in some of the dishes (particularly fermented products like yogurt or kefir) throughout the day. If you are using alternative milk products, ensure they are fortified with B12, vitamin D and calcium.

Drink 6–8 glasses of water through the day; include herbal teas, tea, green tea and coffee if wished.

What to avoid

As this stage of the plan is designed to help you lose weight and help address insulin resistance, it is recommended to avoid alcohol, fruit juice and shop-bought sugary drinks (do not drink your calories, except for protein smoothies, which can be part of a meal).

Avoid white, refined carbohydrates (rice, pasta, breads, crackers, cakes, cookies, crisps, pastries, etc.).

Limit snacks. If you are hungry or particularly active, then include a snack such as a handful of berries or a piece of fruit, a small pot of Greek yogurt or cottage cheese, raw or cooked vegetables, roasted chickpeas or a protein shake.

Keep it simple. There is nothing wrong with keeping your meals simple, especially for breakfast and lunch, if you are short of time. Adherence is key, so keep it easy when it comes to meal planning.

Helpful tips

Use the example meal plans as a guide (see the Appendix). If there are certain foods you don't like, then simply swap them for something similar.

It is important to keep it simple at the start – if you find it easier initially making the same breakfast each day, then fine.

Meal planning and preparation can be helpful when it comes to weight loss. Spend some time at the weekend planning and preparing your meals for the week ahead. Many of the recipes can be made in bulk and frozen.

Be consistent. Weight loss takes time. If you slip up, don't worry – just get back on to the plan and be consistent.

Watch your drinks. If you are a café lover, be mindful that many café drinks are laden with sugar and calories. You would be better switching to black coffee or a drink with a splash of milk, herbal, black or green tea. Remember to drink sufficient water through the day. Add some lemon slices for a little flavour if wished.

MOVING ON – RENEW

The Renew stage of the plan is designed to include a wide range of nutrient-rich dishes to support your health in the long term. Whether you wish to focus more on heart health, bones and joints or brain health, the recipes are rich in nutrients to support long-term health and vitality. Each has a symbol to indicate whether they are beneficial for bone, heart and/or brain health. This may help you personalize your choices according to your individual health goals.

The same principles apply when putting together meals in the Renew stage – you will still wish to ensure sufficient protein-rich foods at each meal and/or snack. Including high-quality protein in every meal can help maintain muscle mass, balance blood sugar levels and reduce cravings, all of which contribute to better energy levels and a healthier metabolism. The Renew recipes are typically higher in fibre-rich carbohydrates – whether from beans and pulses, grains, nuts and seeds or fruits and vegetables. Nourishing fats are also included as they are beneficial for brain and heart health as well as being important in modulating inflammation, which may be more pronounced during menopause. Be mindful of portion sizes, as fats are calorie-dense, but they are a necessary part of a nutritious meal.

Look through the recipes and select those that appeal, aiming for plenty of variety throughout the week.

Brain health

These recipes include nutrients and foods known to support cognition and mood. Examples include omega-3 fatty acids, choline, amino acids, monounsaturated fats, vitamin-, mineral- and antioxidant-rich foods to protect against oxidative stress and support neurotransmitter production, and various antioxidant-rich herbs and spices. Some dishes also include ingredients known for their anti-inflammatory and immune modulation properties (turmeric, green tea, berries, garlic, ginger, mushrooms, fermented foods). Others, such as beetroot, are rich in nitrates to support blood flow and circulation. Probiotic-rich foods (yogurt, kimchi, miso, kefir, sauerkraut, tempeh) to support the gut–brain axis are included. Phytoestrogen-rich foods such as soy, sesame and flaxseed may also be beneficial for brain health and cognition.

Heart health

These recipes tend to be lower in saturated fat, high in fibre, omega-3 fats and monounsaturated fats, and low in added sugar. Foods rich in certain nutrients such as potassium, magnesium and calcium are included to help manage blood pressure, while nitrate-rich foods support blood flow and circulation. A range of foods to lower inflammation (turmeric, oily fish, ginger, garlic, olive oil, avocado) are included, as well as foods to lower high cholesterol such as soy, plant sterols (legumes, nuts, seeds), nuts and seeds, and soluble fibre (e.g., oats, quinoa, beans and pulses, brown rice, mushrooms, apples, pears). A wide variety of colourful fruits and vegetables provide protective antioxidants, fibre and vitamins and minerals to support heart health.

Bone and joint health

These recipes contain key nutrients required for bone health together with a focus on anti-inflammatory foods, such as oily fish and turmeric, which are shown to be beneficial for both joint and bone health. Foods rich in protein and vitamin C to support collagen production are included as well as probiotic-rich foods, which can influence mineral absorption and modulate the immune response. In addition, I have included prebiotic-rich foods to support production of SCFAs, like butyrate, which appear to be beneficial for bone health. Foods high in antioxidants such as vitamins C and E (fruits, vegetables, nuts and seeds, avocado) help to counter the effects of oxidative stress on bone, which, when in excess, can shift the bone remodelling process, increasing bone loss. Recipes rich in phytoestrogens (particularly soy) have also been shown to support bone health.

SUPPLEMENT SUPPORT

It is clear that nutrient status during perimenopause and menopause can influence various health challenges experienced during the transition and long-term health. Maintaining an optimal nutrient status will help reduce the risk of issues such as bone loss, heart disease, blood pressure, blood sugar control and overall vitality. During this stage in life, your nutrient intake needs to support your changing health status and reduce or prevent the risk of certain longer-term health concerns.

To further complicate matters, changes in the gut microbiome and stomach acid production can mean your body becomes less efficient at absorbing nutrients. In addition, with the decline of oestrogen, fundamental changes occur within body systems. Lipid metabolism is altered, your body shifts to a more pro-inflammatory state, and you become less sensitive to insulin and the processes involved in bone health change. Without a conscious effort to ensure your diet is optimized to meet your nutritional needs, there is a risk you will be failing to optimize key levels of certain nutrients. For example, bone-supporting nutrients such as calcium, magnesium and vitamins K and D become increasingly important to slow the bone loss that typically occurs more noticeably around menopause. The use of prescription medicines often increases with age, many of which disrupt nutrient uptakes. For example, proton pump inhibitors, which reduce stomach acidity, can reduce levels of certain minerals like magnesium. Equally the need for certain nutrients may increase. As oestrogens are important for regulating immune function and inflammation, the decline around menopause increases the need for antioxidants such as vitamins A, E and D and omega-3 fatty acids. Lower oestrogen also impacts choline levels, which is crucial for the production of the neurotransmitter acetylcholine involved in memory and mood. Similarly, to support muscle mass, protein becomes increasingly important.

The food matrix, however, is much more than simply individual nutrients. Different components within food work in synergy, and it is the complex different actions and interactions within the food matrix that are particularly beneficial to health. In addition, components such as fibre, which impacts the gut microbiome, can, in turn, impact the absorption and production of certain nutrients for health.

Studies indicate that many of us are failing to achieve optimal levels of important nutrients, which is often confounded by busy lifestyles, eating on the go, following restrictive diets or a reliance on ready meals, all of which can increase the risk of nutritional gaps.[1] This is further exacerbated by the impact that oestrogen and other hormone declines have on the body systems, increasing the demand for certain nutrients.

While taking a multivitamin and multi-mineral is a convenient way to address potential nutritional gaps, you may require a more targeted approach depending on your symptoms, health history and existing diet. Nutrients that may be particularly beneficial include calcium, magnesium, vitamins D and K for bone health, choline, B vitamins and omega-3 fatty acids for both cognitive health and cardiovascular health, probiotics and prebiotics for digestive health, and antioxidant formulas for immune function.

Throughout this book, I have mentioned certain supplemental support for specific concerns or conditions. Please consult a qualified practitioner when considering whether supplements are appropriate for you.

USE OF HORMONE REPLACEMENT THERAPY

HRT is often used to attenuate the undesirable symptoms of menopause by providing exogenous oestrogen (with or without progesterone) to supplement the body's low levels. Studies also indicate HRT has substantial positive impacts beyond menopause symptom relief, such as reducing the risk of osteoporosis and cognitive decline.

Historically, the use of HRT has been surrounded by controversy, largely due to media coverage of the Women's Health Initiative (WHI) studies first published in 2002. The initial findings suggested an increased risk of breast cancer and cardiovascular disease, which led to widespread discontinuation of HRT. However, further analysis has shown that the risks were misinterpreted and overgeneralized. The WHI study population had an older average age (approx. 63 years), meaning findings may not be applicable to women starting HRT earlier. Additionally, the slight increase in breast cancer risk was primarily linked to MPA (medroxy-progesterone acetate), a synthetic progestin. In contrast, oestrogen-only therapy (used in women without a uterus) has been associated with a reduced risk of breast cancer. Today, bioidentical micronized progesterone is used instead of MPA, making the WHI findings less relevant to current HRT protocols.[2]

The age at which HRT is started may be important. Studies suggest that starting HRT within ten years of menopause onset may be most beneficial when it comes to reducing cardiovascular risk and cognitive decline. Starting HRT after ten years of menopause may increase the risk. However, studies do not demonstrate a similar risk in continuing HRT post menopause (when started early). When it comes to HRT, just like many other medications, there are always risks and benefits. What is clear is that the health risks have been overblown, and the potential benefits, whether symptom relief, bone health, psychological or physical wellbeing, are evident. Whether you choose to take HRT, getting the foundations in place when it comes to diet, managing stress, getting quality sleep and sufficient exercise are important for a longer, healthier life.

PART 5

RECIPES

Reset

Renew

Bone health

Brain health

Heart health

Gluten free

Vegetarian

Vegan

BREAKFASTS
Smoothies

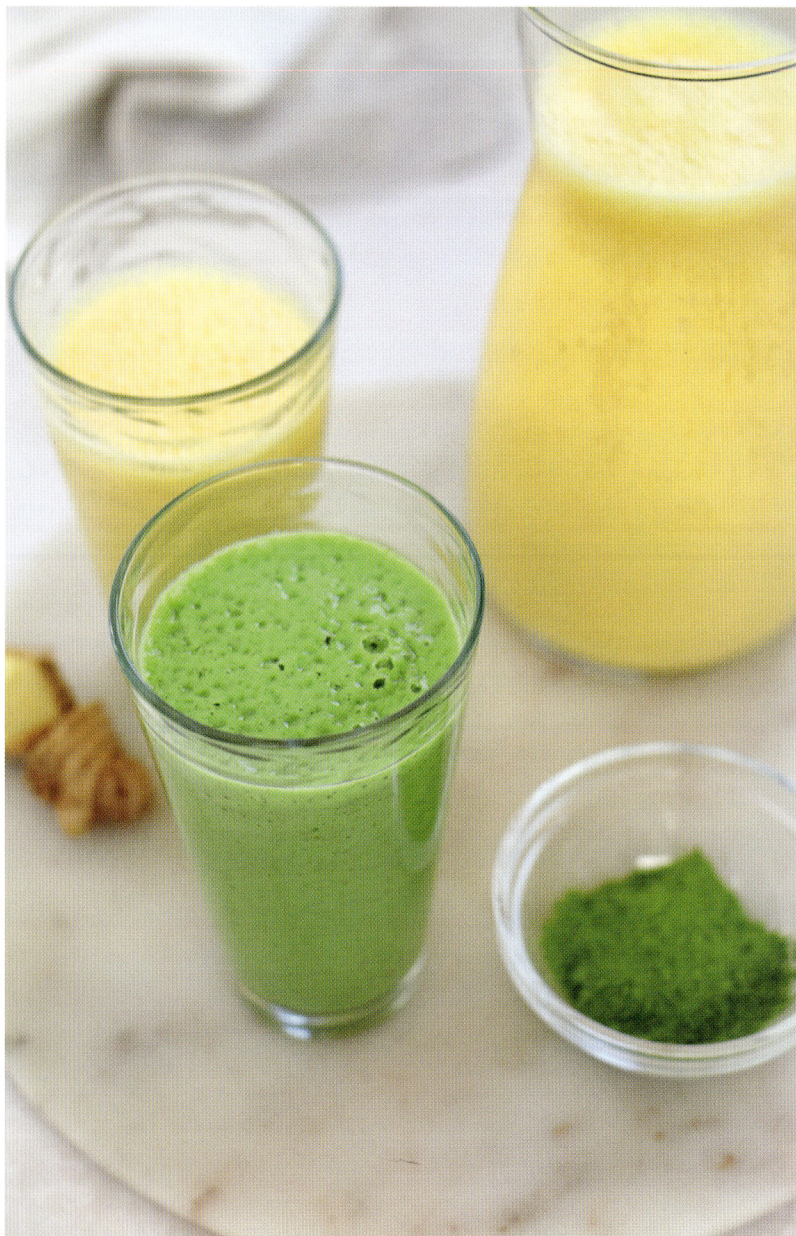

SUPER GREENS SMOOTHIE, TROPICAL IMMUNE BLAST

Blueberry Brain Boost

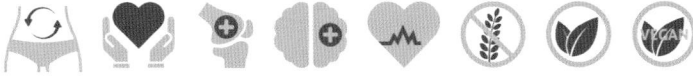

This is packed with antioxidants and nitrates to support brain health. The addition of yogurt provides protein and beneficial microbes to support both your gut and brain. You can swap the Greek yogurt for soy yogurt and use vegan protein powder for a vegan option.

Preparation time: 5 minutes

Serves 2

Ingredients

- 200g frozen blueberries (or a bag of frozen mixed berries)
- 1 small beetroot, cooked
- 150g low-fat Greek yogurt (or soy yogurt)
- 150g coconut water
- 1 ripe pear, cored and chopped
- 1 tbsp shelled hemp seeds
- 30g vanilla protein powder

Method

Place all the ingredients in a high-speed blender and blitz until smooth and creamy. Best served immediately.

Nutrition per serving: 230kcal, Fat 3.4g, of which saturates 0.4g, Carbohydrates 24g, of which sugars 15g, Fibre 5.8g, Protein 23g

Tropical Immune Blast

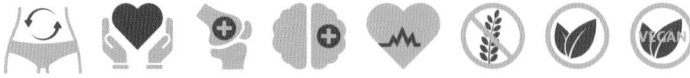

Using kefir provides protein, calcium and probiotics to support the immune system and bone health. This smoothie includes the anti-inflammatory spices ginger and turmeric, as well as pineapple, which is a source of bromelain, a proteolytic enzyme with anti-inflammatory properties. This is an ideal smoothie for joint and bone health, and for supporting the immune system through the winter season.

Preparation time: 5 minutes

Serves 2

Ingredients

- 5g fresh turmeric root, peeled
- 5g fresh ginger, peeled
- 350g pineapple, including core
- 1 large orange, peeled and pips removed
- 200g kefir (or coconut kefir)
- 100g coconut water or water
- 1 tsp ground flaxseed
- Pinch of black pepper
- 30g vegan protein powder

Method

Place all the ingredients in a high-speed blender and blitz until smooth and creamy. Best served immediately.

Nutrition per serving: 243kcal, Fat 4.7g, of which saturates 2.5g, Carbohydrates 27g, of which sugars 25g, Fibre 4.7g, Protein 20g

Super Greens Smoothie

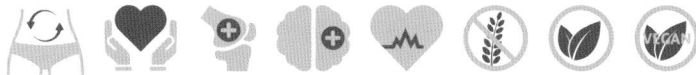

This creamy protein smoothie is light and refreshing, thanks to the addition of coconut water. Adding kiwifruit not only provides fibre and antioxidants, but has also been shown to ease constipation and support better sleep.

Preparation time: 5 minutes

Serves 1

Ingredients

- 1 ripe pear, cored and chopped
- 2 kiwifruit, peeled and chopped
- 125g coconut water
- Handful of spinach leaves
- 3 mint leaves
- 80g silken tofu
- 1 scoop vanilla protein powder
- ½ tsp matcha green tea powder

Method

Place all the ingredients in a high-speed blender and blitz until smooth and creamy. Add a little water to thin, if needed. Best served immediately.

> **Nutrition per serving:** 250kcal, Fat 4.3g, of which saturates 0.9g, Carbohydrates 23g, of which sugars 20g, Fibre 4.1g, Protein 28g

Creamy Chocolate Shake

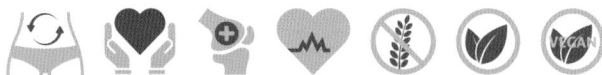

It may seem odd to add cauliflower to a smoothie, but it makes it deliciously creamy. It is also a fabulous way to add more cruciferous vegetables to your diet. Instead of frozen cauliflower florets, you could add leftover cooked cauliflower.

Preparation time: 5 minutes

Serves 2

Ingredients

- 100g frozen cauliflower florets or cauliflower rice (or leftover cooked cauliflower)
- 1 medium-ripe banana
- 1 tsp vanilla extract
- 2 tsp tahini paste
- ½ tsp maca powder
- 2–3 pitted dates, to taste
- 1 scoop chocolate protein powder
- 250ml milk (or soy milk)

Method

Place all the ingredients in a high-speed blender and blitz until smooth and creamy. Best served immediately.

Nutrition per serving: 236kcal, Fat 6.5g, of which saturates 2.5g, Carbohydrates 25g, of which sugars 21g, Fibre 2.7g, Protein 20g

Cinnamon Maca Shake

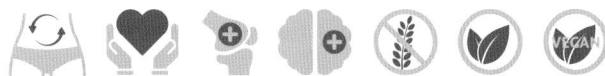

This is a super-easy protein shake. The addition of flaxseed provides fibre and phytoestrogens. Maca is an adaptogenic herb that helps the body adapt to stress, and may also help in alleviating hot flushes and supporting bone health.

Preparation time: 5 minutes

Serves 1

Ingredients

- 250ml milk (or soy milk)
- 1 tsp nut butter
- 1 tsp flaxseed
- 1–2 tsp maca powder, to taste
- 1 tbsp cocoa powder
- ½ tsp ground cinnamon
- 1 scoop chocolate protein powder

Method

Place all the ingredients in a high-speed blender and blitz until smooth and creamy. Best served immediately.

Nutrition per serving: 309kcal, Fat 16g, of which saturates 5.3g, Carbohydrates 8.7g, of which sugars 4g, Fibre 8.2g, Protein 28g

Speedy breakfast ideas

Whether you need something to grab and go or you have a little more time, include a high-protein breakfast to improve your energy levels, reduce cravings later in the day and support muscle mass. Many of the breakfast recipes are quick and easy or can be made ahead or in batches. Here are some additional ideas for when you are short of time.

Scrambled Eggs with Spinach and Salsa

Scramble 2–3 eggs with a handful of spinach and serve with some salsa if wished. You could also add a side of edamame beans for extra fibre, phytoestrogens and protein.

Egg White Omelette with Veggies

Make an omelette with 2–3 egg whites plus 1 whole egg, and fill it with vegetables such as sliced red peppers, tomatoes and mushrooms.

Cottage Cheese with Berries and Seeds

Top 200g low-fat cottage cheese with a handful of mixed berries (such as blueberries or strawberries) and 1 tsp of seeds.

Low-Fat Greek Yogurt with Fruit

Mix 200g 0% fat Greek yogurt with a handful of berries and 1 tbsp of mixed seeds.

Frittata

Bake a frittata (see Oven-Baked Frittata with Roasted Pepper on page 150) using eggs, spinach and cottage cheese. Slice it into wedges for an easy grab-and-go breakfast.

Egg Muffins

To make a tray of egg muffins (about 8), beat together 6 large eggs and season with salt and black pepper. Add chopped leftover vegetables such as broccoli florets or a chopped red pepper and a handful of grated cheese or crumbled feta. Pour the mixture into muffin holes. Bake in the oven for 15–20 minutes (180°C/Gas Mark 4) until they are golden brown and cooked through.

Protein Yogurt with Berries

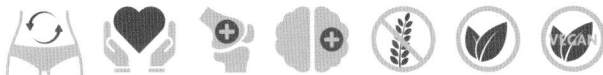

This is a quick and easy high-protein option, ideal for Reset days. Using Greek or soy yogurt is an easy way to add plenty of protein as well as beneficial bacteria for gut health. Berries are a source of polyphenols with prebiotic benefits, making them a perfect pairing with yogurt.

Preparation time: 5 minutes

Serves 1

Ingredients

- 250g 0% fat Greek yogurt (or soy yogurt)
- 1 scoop protein powder, vanilla or chocolate
- 60g fresh berries
- 1 tsp sunflower seeds or other seeds

Method

Mix together the yogurt and protein powder. Top with berries and seeds to serve.

> **Nutrition per serving:** 297kcal, Fat 3.9g, of which saturates 1.5g, Carbohydrates 17g, of which sugars 15g, Fibre 2.3g, Protein 48g

Chocolate Protein Pots

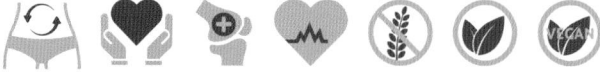

Chocolate for breakfast! Yes please! This is a naturally sweetened protein pot that can be made the night before for ease. It is ideal as a dessert or snack, especially post exercise. For a more indulgent treat, add 30g melted chocolate and blend with the remaining ingredients.

Preparation time: 5 minutes, plus chilling overnight

Serves 1

Ingredients

- 350g silken tofu
- 2–3 tbsp cocoa powder or chocolate protein powder, to taste
- Juice and zest of 1 orange
- Natural yogurt (or soy yogurt), to top

Method

Simply place all the ingredients in a blender and process until smooth. Pour into a glass and chill overnight. Top with a little yogurt to serve.

Nutrition per serving using cocoa powder: 332kcal, Fat 16g, of which saturates 5.1g, Carbohydrates 18g, of which sugars 9.3g, Fibre 9.7g, Protein 24g

---

Nutrition per serving using protein powder: 326kcal, Fat 12g, of which saturates 2.5g, Carbohydrates 17g, of which sugars 11g, Fibre 9.7g, Protein 37g

Creamy Protein Smoothie Bowl

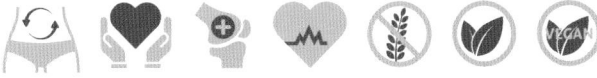

This may sound strange, but the addition of cauliflower adds a wonderful creamy texture. Cauliflower is also a great source of fibre, antioxidants and sulphur-containing compounds that support liver detoxification – important for hormone balance during menopause. Additionally, it contains indole-3-carbinol, which may help with oestrogen metabolism.

Preparation time: 5 minutes

Serves 1

Ingredients

- 30g protein powder, any flavour
- 200g frozen cauliflower rice
- 50g frozen fruit
- Flavourings – 1 tsp vanilla extract and/or ½ tsp cinnamon

Method

Simply place all the ingredients in a blender and process to form a thick smoothie. Spoon or pour into a bowl and serve immediately.

Nutrition per serving: 243kcal, Fat 3.1g, of which saturates 0.7g, Carbohydrates 21g, of which sugars 13g, Fibre 6.1g, Protein 31g

Vanilla Berry Chia Pots

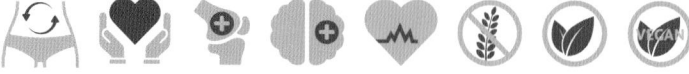

This is a simple high-fibre breakfast option to support digestive health and help keep you feeling full through the morning. Make it the night before to allow time for the chia seeds to soak up the liquid. It is ideal for a grab-and-go breakfast, when time is short in the morning.

Preparation time: 5 minutes

Serves 2

Ingredients

- 200ml semi-skimmed milk (or soy milk)
- 50g Greek yogurt (or soy yogurt)
- 2 tsp honey or maple syrup (optional)
- 1 tsp vanilla extract
- 1 scoop vanilla protein powder
- 50g chia seeds
- 150g frozen or fresh berries

Method

Mix together the milk, half the yogurt, honey or maple syrup, vanilla extract and protein powder. Stir in the chia seeds. Divide the mixture in half and spoon into bowls or glasses or jars.

Place the berries in a pan with a splash of water and simmer for a couple of minutes, mashing them slightly with the back of a wooden spoon. Allow the berries to cool, then spoon half through the chia mixture.

Place the chia mixture and remaining berries in the fridge overnight. In the morning, top the chia mixture with the remaining berry puree and then the remaining yogurt. Serve immediately or keep in the fridge for 1–2 days.

Nutrition per serving: 275g, Fat 11g, of which saturates 2.5g, Carbohydrates 17g, of which sugars 15g, Fibre 12g, Protein 21g

Protein Overnight Oats

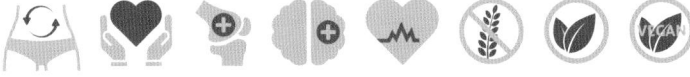

Creamy, packed with protein and fibre, overnight oats are a simple way to start the day. This is a perfect recipe for busy days as it is made the night before. The addition of yogurt gives the oats an extra creamy texture while the protein powder provides plenty of protein to support muscle mass.

Preparation time: 5 minutes, plus overnight

Serves 1

Ingredients

- 30g oats (or gluten-free oats)
- 100ml milk (or soy milk)
- 30g Greek yogurt
  (or soy yogurt)
- 30g protein powder
- 50g blueberries

Method

Simply mix all the ingredients together except for the blueberries. Place in a bowl or Tupperware and chill overnight in the fridge. In the morning, top with the blueberries and serve.

Nutrition per serving: 299kcal, Fat 5.1g, of which saturates 1g, Carbohydrates 26g, of which sugars 6.4g, Fibre 3.8g, Protein 35g

Peanut and Apricot Oat Slice

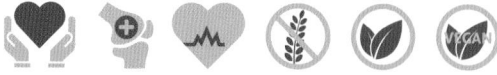

This is a delicious on-the-go slice, loaded with fibre, prebiotics, antioxidants and healthy fats. You can make a batch and keep them in the fridge or freeze them so they're ready to grab if you have a busy day ahead. You can use any nut butter, if wished, to replace the peanut butter.

Preparation time: 15 minutes

Cooking time: 20 minutes

Makes 16 slices

Ingredients

- 150g peanut butter (or other nut butter)
- 50g butter (or dairy-free spread)
- 45g honey or maple syrup
- 1 medium banana, mashed
- 1 egg, beaten
- 160g oats (or gluten-free oats)
- 20g puffed rice
- 1 scoop protein powder or 2 tsp maca powder (optional)
- 50g mixed seeds
- 50g dried apricots, chopped
- 2 tbsp ground flaxseed
- Pinch of salt

Method

Preheat the oven to 180°C/Gas Mark 4. Line a 20cm/8 inch square baking tin with parchment.

Place the peanut butter and butter in a pan and warm gently to melt the butter and soften the peanut butter.

Put all the remaining ingredients in a large bowl and mix well. Add the butter mixture and beat well to ensure the dry ingredients are fully coated. You may wish to use your hands at the end.

Spoon the mixture into the tin and press down firmly. Bake for 20 minutes until golden. Allow to cool completely in the tin and then cut into slices. Store in an airtight container or in the fridge for up to a week.

Nutrition per serving: 177kcal, Fat 10g, of which saturates 3.3g, Carbohydrates 14g, of which sugars 5.1g, Fibre 2.3g, Protein 5.9g

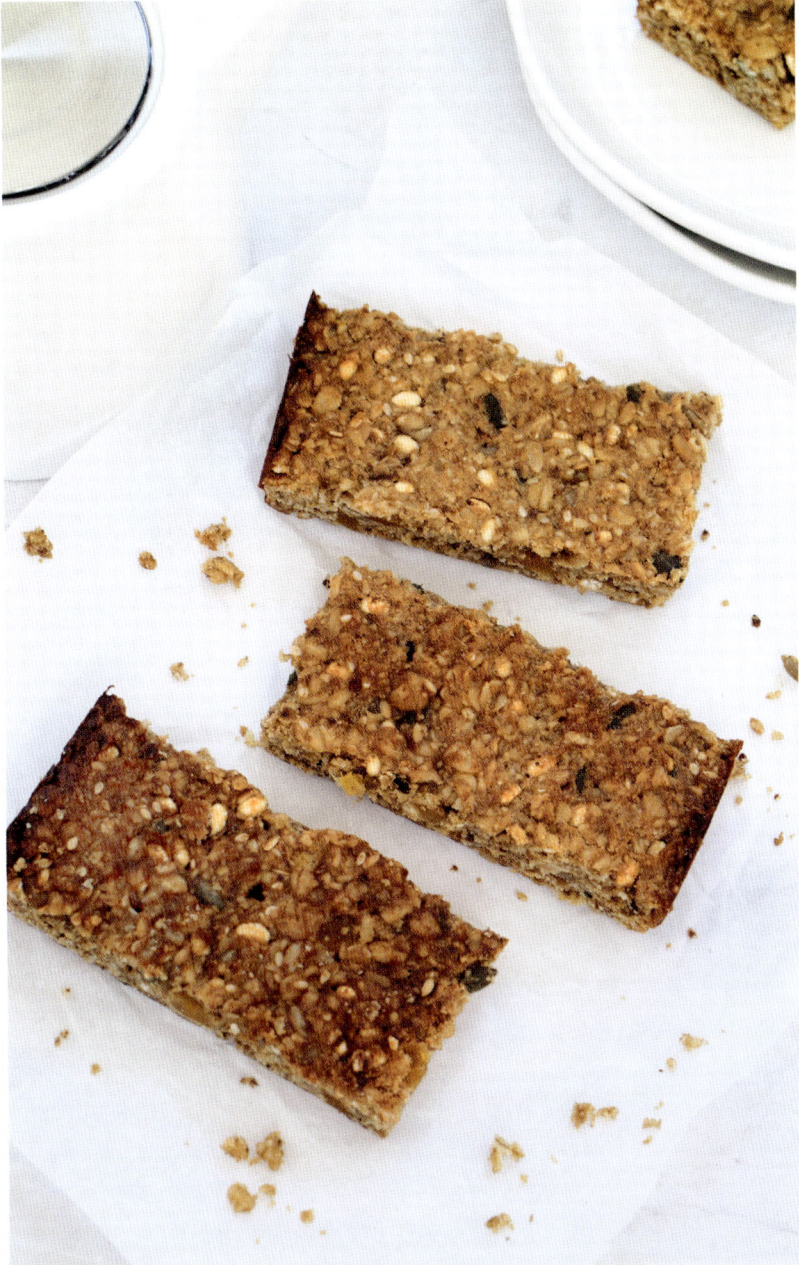

Chai Spiced Granola

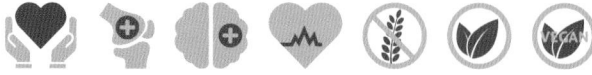

Make this at the weekend ready for those weekdays when time is short. It is delicious as a snack straight from the jar too. Using a range of nuts and seeds provides healthy fats, protein and fibre, plus a good dose of antioxidant vitamin E too.

Preparation time: 15 minutes

Cooking time: 30 minutes

Makes 12 portions

Ingredients

- 125g pecans, chopped
- 125g walnuts, chopped
- 125g mixed seeds
- 2 tbsp whole flaxseed
- 150g oats (or gluten-free oats)
- 2 tsp ground cinnamon
- ½ tsp ground ginger
- ½ tsp ground cloves
- ½ teaspoon sea salt
- 75g goji berries or dried berries

Paste

- 100g pitted soft dates
- 1 orange, peeled and chopped
- 2 tbsp coconut oil, melted
- Scoop of vanilla protein powder (optional)

Method

Preheat the oven to 180°C/Gas Mark 4. Line and lightly grease two baking trays.

Place the nuts, seeds, oats and spices plus the salt in a large bowl and mix well.

Place the dates, orange, coconut oil and protein powder, if using, in a blender and process to form a thick paste. Add a splash of water if needed. Add the date paste to the dry ingredients and mix thoroughly. Use your hands to ensure the ingredients are fully coated in the paste.

Spread out over two baking trays. Place in the oven and bake for 30 minutes, stirring occasionally during cooking. Allow the mix to cool and then stir in the goji berries or dried berries. Store in airtight containers. This will keep for at least a week.

Nutrition per serving: 340kcal, Fat 24g, of which saturates 4.5g, Carbohydrates 21g, of which sugars 9.1g, Fibre 4.7g, Protein 8.2g

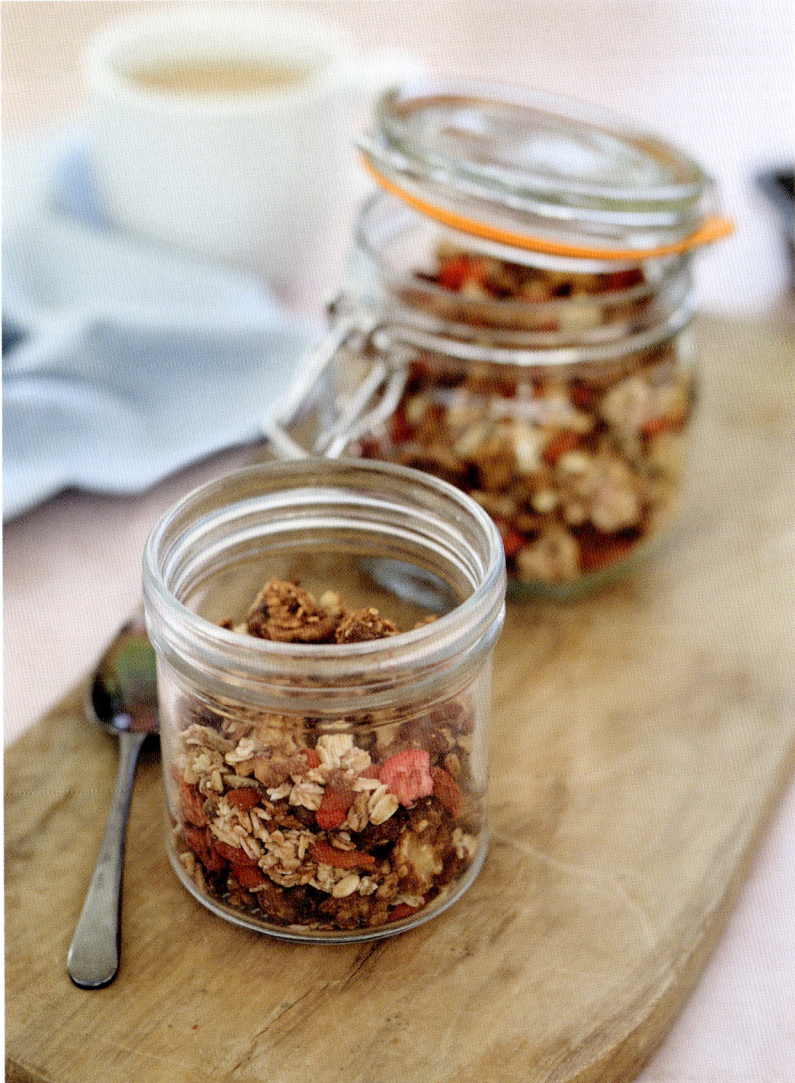

Cottage Cheese Fruit Bowl

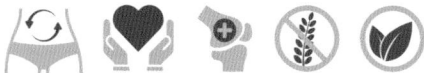

This is a quick and easy breakfast for busy days. It takes minutes to prepare and makes a delicious high-protein option to kick-start the day. Adding nuts or seeds provides additional healthy fats and antioxidants.

Preparation time: 5 minutes

Serves 1

Ingredients

- 200g low-fat cottage cheese
- A pinch of cinnamon (optional)
- 80g fresh berries or 1 apple, chopped
- 30g walnuts, chopped or mixed seeds
- 1 tsp honey or maple syrup (optional)

Method

Put the cottage cheese in a small bowl and mix in the cinnamon, if using. Top with the fruit and scatter over the walnuts or seeds. Drizzle over a little honey or maple syrup, if wished, to serve.

Nutrition per serving: 382kcal, Fat 24g, of which saturates 4.2g, Carbohydrates 14g, of which sugars 14g, Fibre 3.2g, Protein 26g

Buckwheat Pancakes with Blueberry Compote

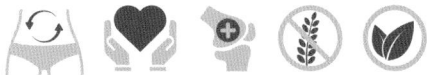

These pancakes provide plenty of fibre, and the addition of cottage cheese gives them an extra protein boost too. For a lighter version use regular flour, or a mixture of buckwheat and regular flour. A gluten-free plain flour mix also works well. Top with a little yogurt and berries for a gut-healthy breakfast treat.

Preparation time: 10 minutes

Cooking time: 10 minutes

Serves 2 (makes around 3–4 pancakes)

Ingredients

- 60g buckwheat flour (or 30g buckwheat and 30g gluten-free or regular plain flour)
- 1 tsp baking powder
- 1 tsp ground flaxseed
- ½ tsp cinnamon
- 130g full-fat cottage cheese
- 1 large egg
- ½ tsp vanilla extract
- 2 tbsp Greek or soy yogurt (to serve)

Berry compote

- 150g fresh or frozen blueberries

Method

To make the berry compote, place the blueberries in a pan with a splash of water and gently cook for 5 minutes until the berries have softened and broken down a little. Stir well as they are cooking. Add a little more water if needed. Set aside. (You could prepare this the night before if wished.)

For the pancakes, simply place all the ingredients in a blender and process until smooth. Heat a pan or griddle to low-medium heat and spray or wipe with a little olive oil. Once hot, pour a little batter into the pan to form small blinis/pancakes. This should make around 3–4 pancakes. Cook until little bubbles form and the edges of the pancakes are solid enough to flip – about 3 minutes.

Cook briefly on the other side. Repeat until all the batter has been used up. Serve with the blueberry compote and yogurt.

Nutrition per serving: 281kcal, Fat 8.2g, of which saturates 3.1g, Carbohydrates 30g, of which sugars 9.1g, Fibre 5.9g, Protein 19g

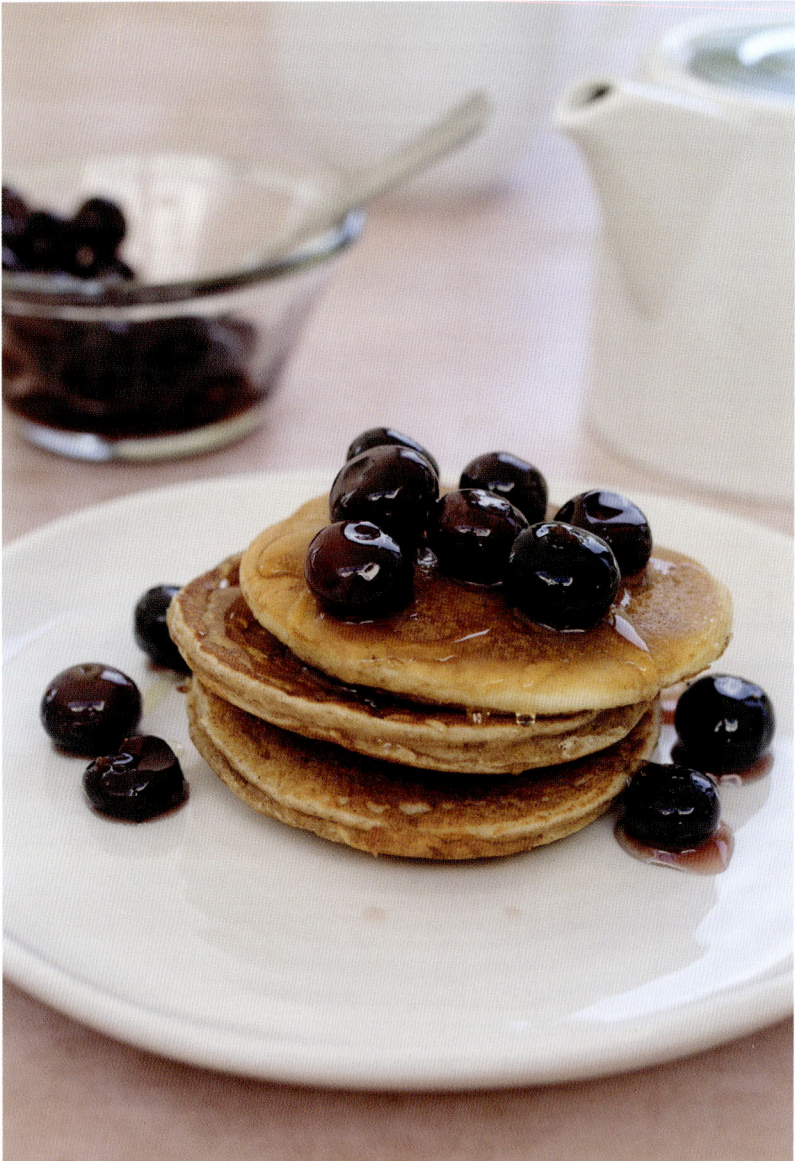

Smashed Edamame Beans with Lemon and Capers

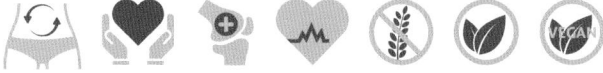

This is a nice alternative to scrambled eggs or tofu. It is also an ideal simple lunch option. It is delicious spread over toasted sourdough, or serve it with some Tomato Flaxseed Crackers.

Preparation time: 10 minutes

Cooking time: 8 minutes

Serves 1

Ingredients

- 150g frozen shelled edamame beans
- 1 tsp olive oil
- 1 garlic clove, crushed (optional)
- 4 cherry tomatoes, halved
- 1 tbsp lemon juice
- 1 tsp capers, drained and roughly chopped
- Salt and pepper to taste
- Chopped fresh herbs – parsley, chives, etc.

To serve: 1 slice wholegrain or sourdough bread or Tomato Flaxseed Crackers (see page 225)

Method

Place the edamame beans in a pan of boiling water. Bring to the boil and simmer for 5 minutes until tender. Drain well.

Heat the oil in a frying pan. Add the edamame beans, garlic (if using) and tomatoes, and stir-fry for 1–2 minutes. Add the lemon juice, capers and salt and pepper to taste. Cook for a further minute, then take off the heat and smash the beans roughly with a fork or potato masher. Serve on toasted bread or accompany with Tomato Flaxseed Crackers.

Nutrition per serving: 328kcal, Fat 13g, of which saturates 1g, Carbohydrates 25g, of which sugars 6.4g, Fibre 11g, Protein 20g

Tofu and Spinach Scramble

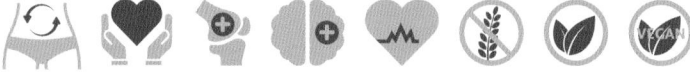

This is one of my favourite breakfast or brunch options. Tofu is a great source of protein, calcium, magnesium and isoflavones – a type of phyto-estrogen that has a mild oestrogenic benefit. Adding nutritional yeast flakes gives the tofu a wonderful slightly cheesy flavour, and provides a good dose of B vitamins too.

Preparation time: 5 minutes

Cooking time: 6 minutes

Serves 2

Ingredients

- 1 tbsp olive oil
- 1 garlic clove, crushed
- 200g cherry tomatoes, halved
- 400g firm tofu, drained
- ¼ tsp ground turmeric
- 2 tbsp nutritional yeast flakes
- 1 tbsp tamari soy sauce
- 2 handfuls of baby spinach or lamb's lettuce
- Salt and black pepper, to taste

To serve: Sourdough or wholegrain toast

Method

Heat the olive oil in a frying pan. Add the garlic and sauté briefly for a minute. Add the tomatoes and heat gently for 2 minutes – just to soften slightly. Add the tofu and turmeric, and use your spatula to break it down into smaller pieces. Cook gently for 2–3 minutes until the excess water has evaporated. Add the nutritional yeast flakes, tamari soy sauce and spinach. Stir gently for a minute to wilt the spinach. Season to taste. Serve on its own or spoon over toasted bread.

Nutrition per serving: 272kcal, Fat 13g, of which saturates 1.9g, Carbohydrates 10g, of which sugars 5g, Fibre 5.1g, Protein 25g

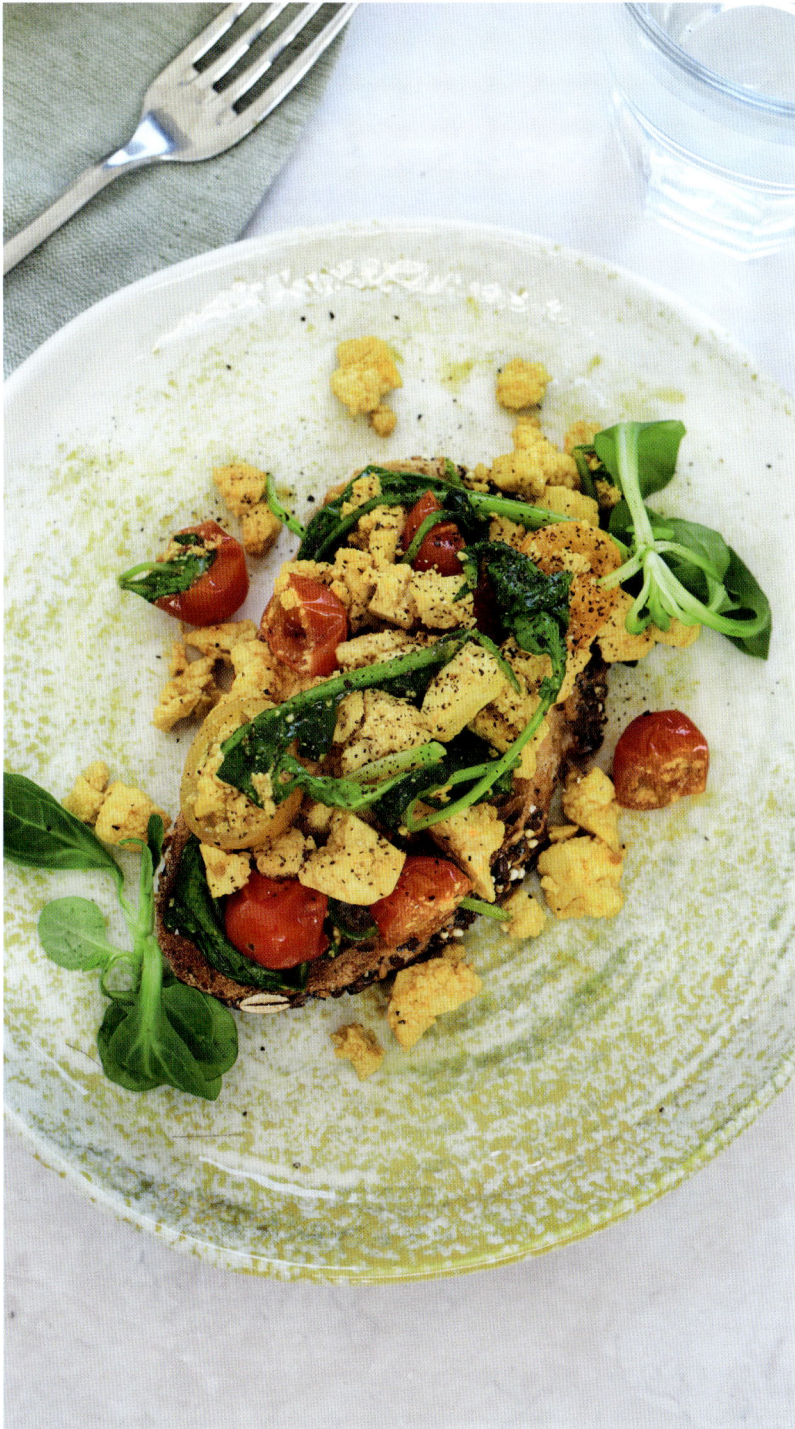

Oven-Baked Frittata with Roast Pepper

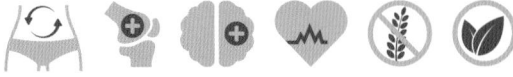

Delicious hot or cold, this makes a perfect grab-and-go breakfast. For a lunch or light dinner option, accompany with a mixed green salad. You can use any leftover vegetables. Using ricotta cheese provides a creamy texture and additional protein too.

Preparation time: 10 minutes

Cooking time: 30–35 minutes

Serves 4

Ingredients

- 2 tsp olive oil
- 1 small red onion, halved and sliced
- 200g baby spinach leaves
- 1 clove garlic, crushed
- 2 roasted red peppers (from a jar), chopped
- 1 tomato, deseeded and diced
- 250g ricotta cheese
- 6 eggs
- 100ml milk
- Salt and pepper to taste

Method

Heat the oven to 220°C/Gas Mark 7.

Heat the oil in a large frying pan and then fry the onion until soft (about 5 minutes). Add the spinach and cook for 3–4 minutes or until wilted. Add the garlic, peppers and tomatoes, cook for 1 minute, and then season. Allow to cool for a few minutes.

Beat the ricotta with the eggs and milk. Season and then stir into the vegetable mixture. Pour into a lightly greased baking dish. Bake for 20–25 minutes until just set in the middle. Cut into squares. Serve hot or cold. This is delicious with a mixed salad.

> **Nutrition per serving:** 442kcal, Fat 28g, of which saturates 14g, Carbohydrates 13g, of which sugars 11g, Fibre 2.3g, Protein 34g

Smoked Salmon with Avocado and Smashed Broad Beans

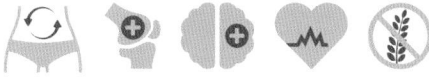

Adding broad beans to the avocado smash is a great way to increase fibre and phytoestrogens. This is quick and simple, and would also make a perfect light lunch with a salad.

Preparation time: 10 minutes

Cooking time: 4 minutes

Serves 2

Ingredients

- 80g frozen (or fresh) broad beans, skinned
- ½ ripe avocado
- 50g Greek yogurt
- Squeeze of lemon juice
- Salt and pepper
- 2 slices rye or sourdough bread (or gluten-free bread)
- 100g smoked salmon
- Sprinkle of whole flaxseed (optional)

Method

Cook the broad beans in boiling water until tender, about 3–4 minutes. Drain. Spoon the avocado into a bowl. Add the beans, yogurt and lemon juice, and mash roughly with a fork. Season with salt and pepper. Toast the bread. Spread the avocado bean smash on the toast and top with the smoked salmon. Sprinkle with flaxseed, if wished.

> **Nutrition per serving:** 315kcal, Fat 13g, of which saturates 2.9g, Carbohydrates 23g, of which sugars 2.2g, Fibre 7.9g, Protein 22g

LUNCH

Mushroom and Herb Omelette with Salsa Verde

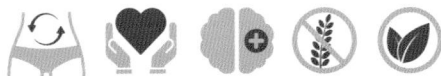

Jazz up your omelette with a drizzle of salsa verde, a fabulous herb dressing, delicious with eggs, meat and fish. Make up a batch and keep it in the fridge for 3–4 days. The addition of egg whites to the omelette is an easy way to increase your overall protein content.

Preparation time: 10 minutes

Cooking time: 6 minutes

Serves 1

Ingredients

- 2 tsp olive oil
- 4 mushrooms, sliced or chopped
- 2 eggs plus 3 egg whites (or a carton of egg whites)
- Handful of chopped fresh herbs, of choice
- Salt and pepper

Salsa verde dressing (save the rest in the fridge – it will keep for 3–4 days)

- Handful of parsley
- Handful of basil leaves
- Handful of mint leaves
- 1 garlic clove, crushed
- 1 tbsp lemon juice
- 1 anchovy, chopped
- 1 tbsp capers
- 1 tbsp red wine vinegar
- ½ tsp Dijon mustard
- 3 tbsp olive oil
- Sea salt and pepper to taste

Method

In a blender or food processor add all the salsa verde ingredients and process to form a chunky paste – add a dash of water to help blend if needed. Taste and season as needed. Place in the fridge until required.

Heat the oil in a frying pan and sauté the mushrooms for 1–2 minutes until soft.

Beat together the egg and egg whites. Season with salt and pepper and add the herbs. Pour the egg mixture into the pan and swirl around. Cook for a minute to let the egg start to set. Use a spatula to pull the egg into the centre and tip the pan to allow any uncooked egg to flow into the space. Continue until the egg has almost all set.

Turn out and serve with a little of the salsa verde. Accompany with a large mixed salad.

> **Nutrition per serving with 1 tbsp salsa verde:** 327kcal, Fat 24g, of which saturates 4.8g, Carbohydrates 2.3g, of which sugars 0.5g, Fibre 0.8g, Protein 27g

LUNCH

Korean Rolled Omelette

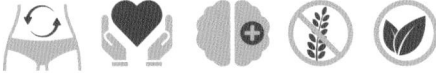

This rolled egg recipe is filled with mushrooms, onion and chilli, and makes a delicious protein-packed lunch, ideal for lunch boxes. You could use any leftover vegetables.

Preparation time: 15 minutes

Cooking time: 15 minutes

Serves 2

Ingredients

- 5 eggs plus 2 egg whites
- Pinch of salt and black pepper
- 1 tbsp whole milk
- ½ tsp apple cider vinegar
- Olive oil, for greasing pan
- 1 spring onion, finely chopped
- 4 shiitake mushrooms, diced
- 1 red chilli, deseeded and diced
- ¼ red pepper, diced
- 1 tbsp chives, chopped

Method

Whisk the eggs, salt, pepper, milk and vinegar in a medium bowl until well combined and smooth. Pour the egg mixture through a sieve or fine mesh strainer into a clean bowl. This helps make the texture of the egg roll smooth and easier to roll.

Add 1 tsp of olive oil to a non-stick frying pan. When hot, add the vegetables and season, and cook, stirring well over a medium-high heat until tender – about 3 minutes. Remove the vegetables from the pan. Add to the egg mixture and mix well. In the same frying pan, add a little more olive oil.

Add a third of the egg-veggie mixture and swirl the pan gently to evenly distribute them. Let the mixture cook for 4 minutes until the eggs start to set. Use a spatula to start to roll the egg in towards the centre. Leave the far side flat and unrolled. Slide the egg roll to the far side of the pan and, if needed, add a little more oil to the empty side of the pan.

LUNCH

Add half the remaining egg-veggie mixture to the empty side of the pan and gently swirl it around to even it out. Repeat the same process: let the egg cook for 3–4 minutes, and when it is set, with only a bit of moisture left in the middle, roll the omelette three-quarters of the way up and slide it to the far side of the pan. Repeat the process using the remaining egg mixture. Once cooked, roll up all the way.

Remove the egg roll from the pan and let it rest on a cutting board for a few minutes. When it's cool enough to handle, slice the egg roll into 5cm/2 inch pieces and serve hot or cold. The egg roll will last in the refrigerator for 2–3 days in an airtight container.

Nutrition per serving: 235kcal, Fat 13g, of which saturates 3.8g, Carbohydrates 4g, of which sugars 2g, Fibre 1.1g, Protein 20g

LUNCH

Tofu Burrito

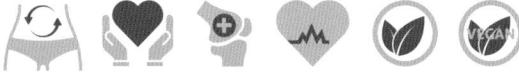

This is a quick and easy grab-and-go meal that can made in advance and reheated if wished. You can also prepare the filling in a bigger batch and keep it in the fridge for 2–3 days to use as a filling, or it is delicious on its own with a salad.

Preparation time: 10 minutes

Cooking time: 10 minutes

Serves 1

Ingredients

- 1 tsp olive oil
- 150g firm tofu, crumbled
- 1 tbsp tamari soy sauce
- 1 tbsp nutritional yeast flakes
- Salt and pepper
- 1 garlic clove, crushed
- 1 tsp smoked paprika
- 1 tsp cumin powder
- 1 tsp onion powder
- Pinch chilli flakes
- 1 tbsp tomato puree

To serve: 1 small wholegrain wrap, shredded lettuce, 1 tomato, chopped, 2 tsp mayonnaise or guacamole (optional)

Method

Heat the oil in a large frying pan. Add the tofu and stir-fry for a couple of minutes, to lightly brown. Add the remaining ingredients and sauté gently for 3–4 minutes. The mixture should be dry.

If using, spread a little mayonnaise or guacamole in the centre of the wrap. Pile the tofu mixture along the centre and scatter over lettuce and tomato, as wished. Fold over the ends to form a parcel.

Heat the frying pan to a medium heat. Place the burrito fold-side down in the pan and cook briefly on each side until lightly golden. Slice in half to serve.

Nutrition per serving: 403kcal, Fat 20g, of which saturates 3.1g, Carbohydrates 27g, of which sugars 5.6g, Fibre 7g, Protein 24g

LUNCH

LUNCH
Soups

Sweet Potato Soup with Ginger and Apple

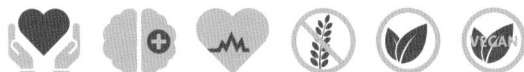

This is a vibrant soup packed with antioxidants vitamins A and C, making it ideal for skin health, plus fibre to support a healthy gut. Adding turmeric can help calm inflammation in the body. You can make a batch of this soup and freeze it in portions for ease. For a Reset meal, accompany with protein on the side, such as 100g cooked chicken, cooked tofu or tempeh, with a side salad.

Preparation time: 15 minutes

Cooking time: 20 minutes

Serves 4

Ingredients

- 1 tbsp olive oil
- 1 medium onion, diced
- 4 garlic cloves, peeled and chopped
- 2.5cm/1 inch fresh ginger, chopped
- 1 sweet potato, peeled and diced (about 300g)
- 2 carrots, chopped
- 2 tsp ground turmeric
- 1 apple chopped
- Sea salt and black pepper
- 800ml vegetable or chicken stock
- 1 can butterbeans, drained
- 1 tbsp lime juice

To serve: Chopped parsley

Method
Add the oil to a large pot over a medium-high heat. When hot, add the onion and let it cook for 3–4 minutes. Add the garlic and ginger and cook for 1

more minute. Add the sweet potato, carrots, turmeric and chopped apple, season with sea salt and black pepper, and stir the pot for about 30 seconds.

Add the stock to the pot and bring to a boil. Reduce the heat to medium and simmer for 12–15 minutes, or until the vegetables are soft.

Add the butterbeans and then transfer the soup to a blender and blend until smooth. Pour the soup back into the pot, add the lime juice and heat through. Serve with the chopped parsley sprinkled on top.

Nutrition per serving: 230kcal, Fat 4.3g, of which saturates 0.7g, Carbohydrates 36g, of which sugars 17g, Fibre 11g, Protein 5.8g

LUNCH
Soups

Tom Yum Soup

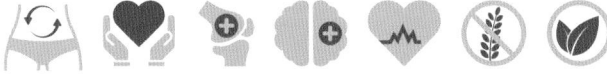

This is a lighter version of a classic Thai dish that is made using tofu, mushrooms and pak choi. The combination of spices can be beneficial for immune health, while the addition of tofu provides protein and phytoestrogens that are useful for calming hot flushes.

Preparation time: 15 minutes

Cooking time: 25 minutes

Serves 4

Ingredients

- 2 lemongrass stalks
- 1 tbsp olive oil
- 1 tsp chopped ginger
- 1 onion, diced
- 4 cloves garlic, minced
- 2 red chillies, deseeded and chopped
- 800ml vegetable stock
- 2–3 tsp tom yum paste
- 4 kaffir lime leaves (optional)
- 2 tbsp lime juice
- 2 tbsp tamari soy sauce
- 2 tsp brown sugar or coconut sugar
- 1 tsp fish sauce (optional)
- 1 x 400g can chopped tomatoes
- 200ml canned light coconut milk
- 400g firm tofu, dried, then cut into cubes
- 6 shiitake mushrooms, sliced
- Handful of sugar snap peas or mangetout
- 2 pak choi, cut into large pieces or halved, if small

To serve: Fresh coriander leaves, chopped

Method

Trim the lemongrass stalks and discard the outer leaves. Use the back of your knife to bash each stalk (this helps release the oils). Cut each stalk in half. Heat the oil in a large saucepan. Add the lemongrass and sauté for 1 minute until fragrant, and then add the ginger, onion, garlic and chillies, and sauté for 2–3 minutes.

Add the stock, tom yum paste and lime leaves and bring to a boil. Reduce the heat to a low simmer and cover. Cook for about 10 minutes to allow the flavours to develop. Add the lime juice, tamari soy sauce, sugar and fish sauce (if using), chopped tomatoes and coconut milk, and heat through.

Add the tofu, mushrooms, sugar snap peas and pak choi to the pan and simmer uncovered for 5 minutes. Remove the lemongrass stalks. Spoon into bowls and garnish with coriander leaves.

Nutrition per serving: 210kcal, Fat 9.1g, of which saturates 3.9g, Carbohydrates 16g, of which sugars 10g, Fibre 3.3g, Protein 14g

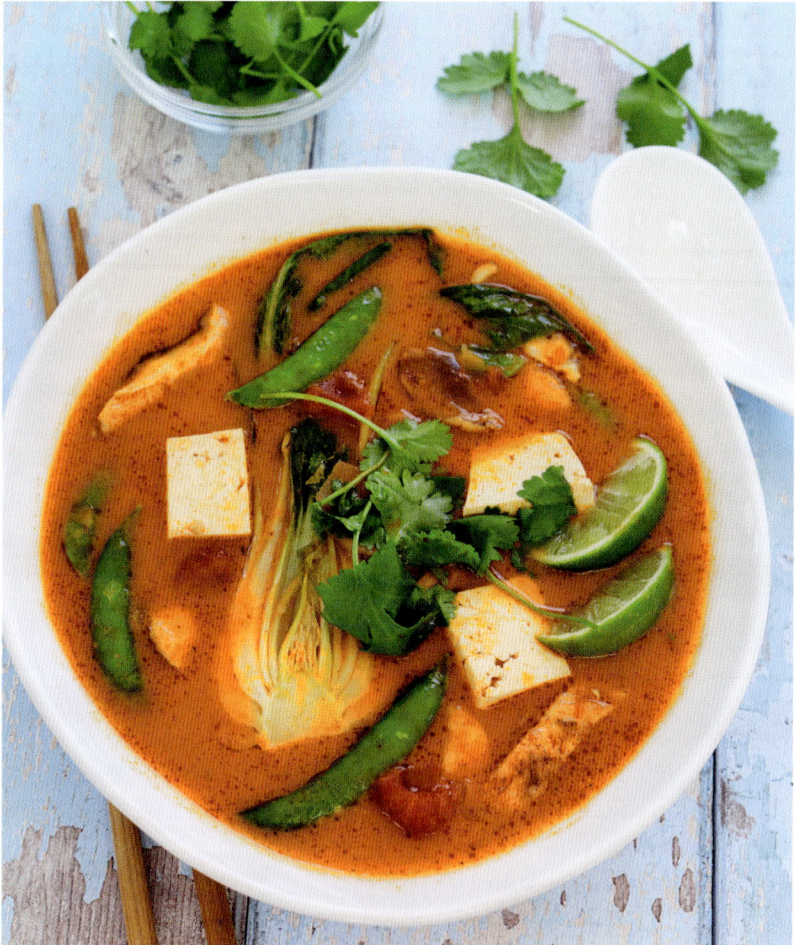

Roasted Broccoli and Fennel Soup

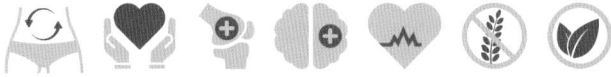

This is a beautiful and light yet creamy-tasting soup. Broccoli contains compounds such as kaempferol, known to lower inflammation in the body, as well as providing antioxidants and fibre. Cruciferous vegetables like broccoli have a positive impact on the metabolism of oestrogen, lowering the metabolites linked to an increased risk of certain cancers. Blending in silken tofu not only creates a lovely creamy texture but provides plenty of protein, calcium and phytoestrogens too.

Preparation time: 5 minutes

Cooking time: 30 minutes

Serves 4

Ingredients

- 300g broccoli, chopped
- 2 fennel bulbs, chopped
- 1 tbsp olive oil
- 1 onion, chopped
- 2 garlic cloves, chopped
- 1 litre vegetable stock
- 1 pear, cored and chopped
- 300g silken tofu

To serve: 30g toasted mixed seeds

Method

Preheat the oven to 200°C/Gas Mark 6.

Place the broccoli and fennel in a baking dish and drizzle over half the olive oil and toss well. Bake in the oven for around 20 minutes, until lightly golden.

Heat the remaining olive oil in a large pan and sauté the onion and garlic for a couple of minutes. Add the broccoli, fennel and vegetable stock and bring to a boil. Simmer for 5–10 minutes.

Place the soup in a blender with the pear and silken tofu and blitz until creamy. Pour back into the pan and warm through. Spoon into bowls and scatter with toasted seeds.

> **Nutrition per serving:** 212kcal, Fat 9.5g, of which saturates 1.4g, Carbohydrates 18g, of which sugars 12g, Fibre 7.8g, Protein 10g

LUNCH
Soups

Minestrone Soup

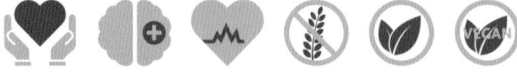

This is a hearty, chunky soup, packed with an array of nutrient-rich vegetables. The addition of beans provides protein and fibre, which can help keep you feeling fuller for longer.

Preparation time: 10 minutes

Cooking time: 35 minutes

Serves 4

Ingredients

- 1 tbsp olive oil
- 1 onion, finely chopped
- 2 carrots, roughly diced
- 2 sticks celery, chopped
- 1 courgette, roughly chopped
- 1 leek, shredded
- 1 small potato, peeled and cut into dice (150g)
- 2 garlic cloves, crushed
- 1 tsp smoked paprika
- 2 x 400g cans chopped tomatoes
- 300ml chicken or vegetable stock
- 200g (¼) Savoy cabbage, shredded
- 1 x 400g can cannellini beans, drained and rinsed
- Sea salt and black pepper, to taste

To serve: 1 tbsp chopped parsley

Method

Heat the oil in a large saucepan and sauté the onion, carrots, celery, courgette, leek and potato over a low heat for about 15 minutes. Add the garlic and paprika, and sauté for another 5 minutes, stirring all the time. Add the chopped tomatoes and stock. Simmer for 15 minutes.

Add the cabbage and beans and cook for a further 5 minutes. Season to taste. Divide the soup between bowls. Drizzle with a little olive oil and top with chopped parsley.

Nutrition per serving: 236kcal, Fat 4.3g, of which saturates 0.7g, Carbohydrates 34g, of which sugars 20g, Fibre 11g, Protein 8.3g

Pan-Fried Tempeh with Sweet Soy Ginger Dressing

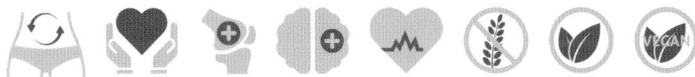

This is a colourful salad packed with antioxidants, vitamins and minerals and tossed with a tangy dressing. Tempeh is fermented soy and rich in protein and isoflavones to ease hot flushes and support bone health. Instead of frying the tempeh, you could air-fry it until lightly golden.

Preparation time: 15 minutes

Cooking time: 7 minutes

Serves 2

Ingredients

- 200g tempeh, bite-size pieces
- 1 tbsp tamari soy sauce
- 1 tbsp nutritional yeast flakes
- 1 tbsp olive oil

For the salad

- 200g sprouting broccoli or regular broccoli, cut into small florets
- 100g sugar snap peas or green beans
- Large handful of lettuce leaves, shredded
- ¼ cucumber, deseeded and diced
- ½ red pepper, cored, deseeded and cut into chunks

Dressing

- 5 tbsp tamari soy sauce
- 1 tbsp honey or maple syrup
- 1 red chilli, deseeded and chopped
- 2 garlic cloves, crushed
- 1 tbsp ginger, finely chopped
- Juice of 2 limes
- 1 tbsp rice vinegar

To serve: 1 tbsp sesame seeds

Method

Place the tempeh in a bowl and drizzle over the tamari soy sauce and nutritional yeast flakes. Toss well and set aside for 5 minutes.

Make up the dressing by whisking all the ingredients together.

Cook the broccoli and sugar snap peas in boiling water until al dente – about 2–3 minutes. Drain and immerse immediately in cold water. Drain again.

Heat the oil in a large sauté pan and cook the tempeh until golden on all sides, about 3–4 minutes. Alternatively air-fry for around 5 minutes until lightly golden.

Place the vegetables in a large bowl and add the tempeh. Pour over the dressing and toss together well. Sprinkle with sesame seeds and serve.

Nutrition per serving: 390kcal, Fat 14g, of which saturates 2.6g, Carbohydrates 24g, of which sugars 15g, Fibre 12g, Protein 32g

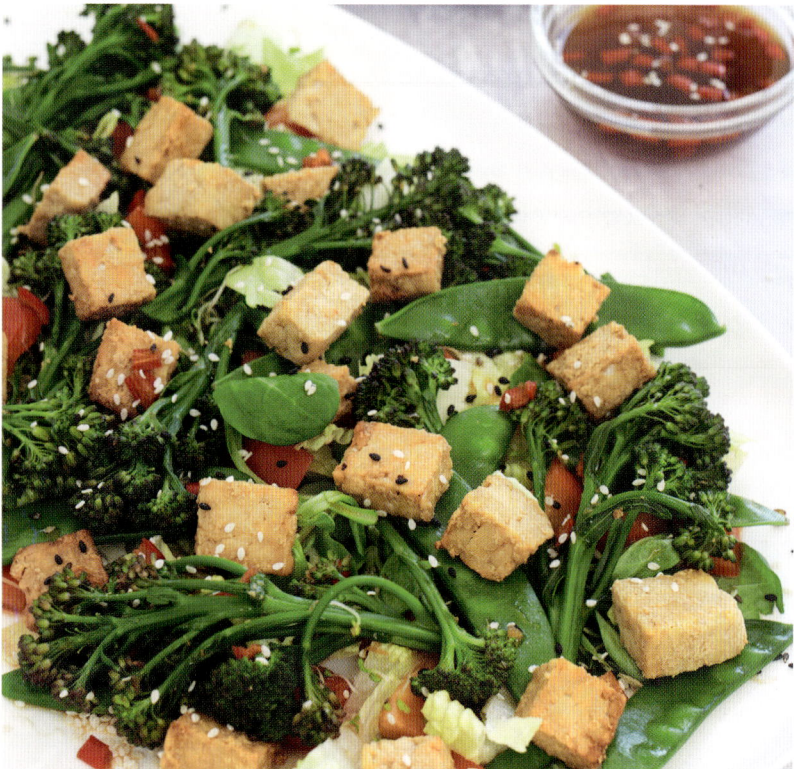

Creamy Kale Salad with Chopped Apple

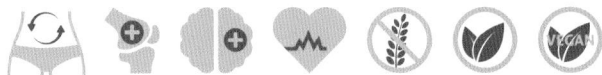

This is a delicious, creamy salad, packed with antioxidants and bone health nutrients like calcium, magnesium and vitamin K. It can be prepared in advance and kept in the fridge for 2–3 days. Accompany with a protein of your choice (e.g., cooked mackerel, chicken, tofu).

Preparation time: 15 minutes

Serves 2

Ingredients

- 300g kale
- ½ tsp sea salt
- 1 tbsp nutritional yeast flakes
- 6 cherry tomatoes, halved
- 1 apple, finely diced
- 1 roasted pepper (from a jar), chopped

Dressing

- 2 tbsp tahini
- 2 tbsp lemon juice
- 2 tsp maple syrup or honey
- 1 tsp tamari soy sauce
- 2 tbsp water
- 1 tbsp nutritional yeast flakes

Method

Place all the ingredients for the dressing in a blender or food processor and blend until creamy.

Remove any tough stems from the kale, chop and place in a large bowl. Add a pinch of salt and nutritional yeast flakes and massage the kale with your hands until the leaves begin to wilt. Add the dressing and mix everything well. Toss in the tomatoes, apple and pepper. Serve with additional protein of your choice, if wished.

> **Nutrition per serving::** 338kcal, Fat 14g, of which saturates 2.1g, Carbohydrates 29g, of which sugars 27g, Fibre 13g, Protein 17g

Sicilian Courgette Salad with Feta

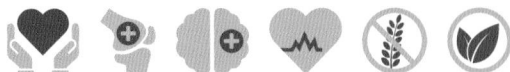

This Mediterranean-inspired salad is light and tangy. Here courgettes are spiralized and tossed with an array of antioxidant-rich vegetables in a lemon and herb dressing. Adding the feta provides plenty of calcium and protein.

Preparation time: 15 minutes

Serves 2

Ingredients

- 3 medium courgettes
- 1 tsp olive oil
- ½ red onion, chopped
- ½ tsp ground cumin
- Pinch of sea salt
- 12 cherry tomatoes, halved

- 2 tsp capers, rinsed
- ½ can drained chickpeas or butterbeans
- 80g low-fat feta cheese, crumbled

Dressing

- Juice of ½ lemon
- 1 tbsp olive oil
- Handful of parsley, chopped
- Handful of mint, chopped

- Handful of coriander leaves
- 1 preserved lemon (flesh and seeds discarded), chopped

Method

Using a spiralizer, create long noodles from the courgettes, or use a swivel potato peeler to create long strands. Place in a bowl.

Heat the oil and sauté the onion with the cumin and a pinch of salt for 2 minutes, then add the cherry tomatoes and sauté for a further minute, to soften very slightly.

To make the dressing place all the ingredients in a food processor and blitz to combine.

Put the onion, tomatoes, capers and chickpeas in the bowl with the courgettes. Pour over the lemon and herb dressing and lightly toss. Scatter over the feta to serve.

Nutrition per serving: 310kcal, Fat 15g, of which saturates 4.5g, Carbohydrates 21g, of which sugars 10g, Fibre 5.6g, Protein 17g,

LUNCH
Salads

Lemon and Herb Quinoa Bowl

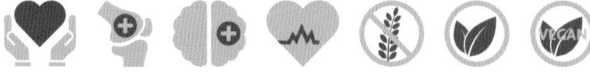

This is the taste of the Middle East. The dish is packed with fresh herbs for flavour and antioxidants. I have used quinoa for its distinctive nutty flavour, but you could substitute with brown rice or millet instead. The addition of chickpeas is a great way to add protein, fibre and phytoestrogens. Serve on its own, or for a higher-protein option, accompany with a piece of fish, chicken or cooked tempeh.

Preparation time: 10 minutes

Cooking time: 30 minutes

Serves 4

Ingredients

- 150g quinoa, millet or brown rice
- 350ml vegetable stock
- 1 tsp cumin seeds
- 80ml olive oil
- 1 red onion, finely chopped
- Juice and zest of 2 lemons
- ¼ tsp ground cumin
- ¼ tsp ground coriander
- ¼ tsp cinnamon
- Pinch of salt
- 1 cucumber, deseeded and diced
- 4 tomatoes, deseeded and diced
- 1 roasted pepper (from a jar), drained and sliced
- 2 large handfuls of parsley, finely chopped
- Large handful of mint, finely chopped
- 1 preserved lemon (flesh and seeds discarded), finely chopped
- 1 x 400g can chickpeas, drained

Method

Place the quinoa in a small pan and add the vegetable stock. Bring to a boil, cover and simmer for 15 minutes. Turn off the heat and leave the quinoa to steam (lid covered) for 5–10 minutes. Cool.

Heat a frying pan and dry toast the cumin seeds briefly, until lightly golden. Remove from the pan. Add a dash of oil and the onion. Fry for 5 minutes until the onion is softened.

Mix the remaining olive oil with the lemon juice and spices. Place the quinoa in a bowl and toss in the remaining ingredients. Season to taste.

Nutrition per serving: 470kcal, Fat 29g, of which saturates 4.4g, Carbohydrates 38g, of which sugars 4.7g, Fibre 5.1g, Protein 10g

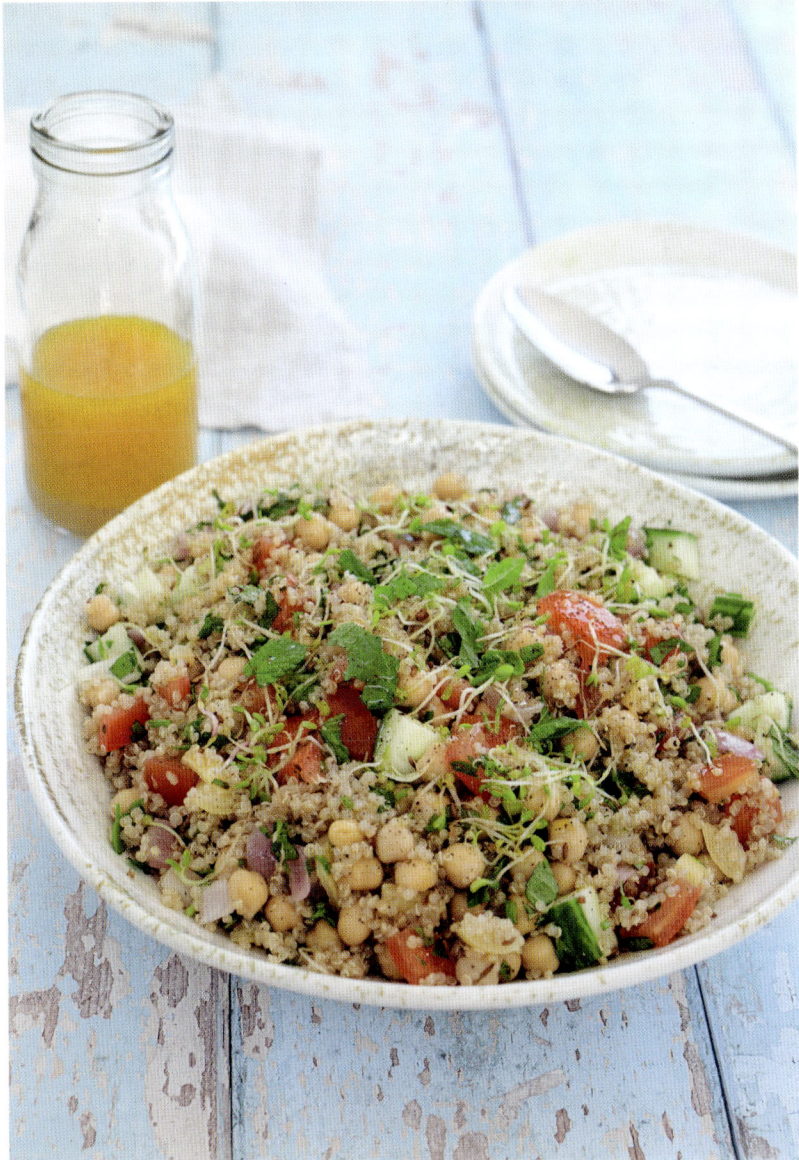

Mixed Bean, Roasted Red Pepper Salad with Sherry Vinegar Dressing

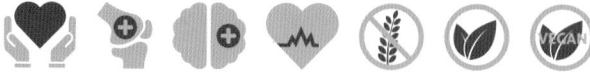

This is a quick and easy lunch using mainly store cupboard ingredients, and it is robust enough for a packed lunch. Being loaded with antioxidants, isoflavones, protein and fibre, beans are an ideal food during menopause.

Preparation time: 15 minutes

Serves 2

LUNCH Salads

Ingredients

- 1 x 400g can butterbeans, drained and rinsed
- 1 x 400g can cannellini beans, drained and rinsed
- 2 roasted red peppers (from a jar), drained and cut into chunks
- ½ red onion, finely diced
- ½ cucumber, deseeded and diced
- 100g cherry tomatoes, halved
- 1 stalk celery, finely chopped
- 100g lambs' lettuce or baby spinach leaves
- Large handful of parsley, chopped

Dressing

- 1 tbsp sherry vinegar
- 2 tbsp extra virgin olive oil
- ¼ tsp Dijon mustard
- Pinch of sugar
- Salt and black pepper, to taste

Method

Make up the dressing by whisking all the ingredients together in a small bowl.

Place all the ingredients for the salad in a bowl and mix gently. Drizzle over the dressing and toss lightly.

Nutrition per serving: 406kcal, Fat 15g, of which saturates 2.5g, Carbohydrates 41g, of which sugars 16g, Fibre 18g, Protein 16g

Roasted Vegetables and Puy Lentils with Harissa Dressing

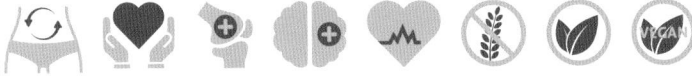

A vibrant, warming dish packed with antioxidants and fibre to support the gut microbiome and balance blood sugar. The harissa dressing adds a flavourful kick to the lentils.

Preparation time:

Cooking time:

Serves 2

Ingredients

- 1 sweet potato, peeled and cut into chunks (250g)
- 1 red onion, cut into large chunks
- 1 red pepper, deseeded and cut into chunks
- 1 yellow pepper, deseeded and cut into chunks
- Salt and pepper
- 200g baby spinach leaves
- 250g cooked puy lentils (from a can or pouch)
- Handful of coriander, chopped

Dressing

- 2 tbsp olive oil
- 1 tsp harissa
- ¼ tsp ground cumin
- 1 tbsp lemon juice
- Pinch of sugar
- Salt and pepper

Method

Preheat the oven to 200°C/Gas Mark 6.

Arrange the sweet potato, onion and peppers on a roasting tray and season. Whisk all the dressing ingredients together. Pour half over the vegetables and mix. Roast in the oven for 30–40 minutes until tender. Remove from the oven and stir in the spinach leaves.

LUNCH
Salads

Pour over the remaining dressing and mix well. Season to taste and scatter with the coriander to serve. Can be served hot or cold.

Nutrition per serving: 500kcal, Fat 16g, of which saturates 2.4g, Carbohydrates 61g, of which sugars 17g, Fibre 16g, Protein 19g

Teriyaki Chicken Noodle Salad

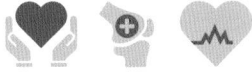

This Asian noodle salad is bursting with fiery flavours, crunchy veg, nutty sesame seeds and griddled chicken. It is packed with antioxidants, protein and fibre, creating an energizing and filling salad.

Preparation time: 15 minutes

Marinating time: 30 minutes

Cooking time: 10 minutes

Serves 2

Ingredients

- 2 chicken breasts, cut into chunks
- 4 tbsp teriyaki sauce
- 4 tsp tamari soy sauce
- 1 tsp olive oil
- 100g udon, soba or flat rice noodles
- 100g tenderstem broccoli, chopped small
- 100g green beans, trimmed and halved
- 1 spring onion, thinly sliced
- 1 tsp sesame oil
- 1 tsp rice wine vinegar
- 60g edamame beans, cooked
- ½ red chilli, deseeded and diced

To serve: Sesame seeds

Method

Place the chicken breasts between two pieces of cling film and bash lightly to flatten into thin escalopes – this will make cooking quicker. Place the chicken in a shallow container and drizzle over 2 tbsp of the teriyaki sauce and 2 tsp of the tamari soy sauce and 1 tsp olive oil. Marinate in the fridge for 30 minutes.

Cook the noodles according to the packet instructions. About 3 minutes before the end of cooking add the broccoli and beans. Drain and refresh under a cold tap.

Heat a griddle pan until medium hot. Griddle the pieces of chicken on each side, about 3–4 minutes until cooked through. Alternatively, you can place them under a grill and cook for 6–8 minutes, turning halfway through. Slice each chicken breast.

Mix the remaining teriyaki sauce and tamari soy sauce with the sesame oil and rice wine vinegar. Toss the noodles together with all the vegetables, including the edamame beans and chilli. Pour over the sauce and toss lightly. Top with the chicken and scatter with a few sesame seeds to serve.

Nutrition per serving: 445kcal, Fat 7.9g, of which saturates 1.2g, Carbohydrates 49g, of which sugars 13g, Fibre 7.2g, Protein 41g

Chicken Panzanella Salad

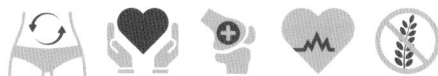

This salad is light and fresh-tasting, and delicious served warm or cold. Poaching the chicken keeps it wonderfully moist and allows you to shred it easily.

Preparation time: 15 minutes

Cooking time: 28 minutes

Serves 2

Ingredients

- 2 chicken breasts
- 1 pitta bread, torn into small pieces (or gluten free pitta bread)
- 1 red pepper, cut into chunks
- 250g cherry tomatoes, halved
- ½ red onion, chopped
- 1 celery stalk, sliced
- 6 olives, pitted and halved
- 1 tbsp capers rinsed
- ½ cucumber, deseeded and sliced
- Handful of basil, shredded
- Handful of parsley, chopped
- 2 tbsp olive oil
- 1 tbsp balsamic vinegar
- 1 garlic clove, crushed
- Salt and pepper to taste

Method

Place the chicken breasts in a pan and cover with water. Bring to the boil, then cover and simmer for 15 minutes. Turn off the heat and allow the chicken to sit in the water for a further 5 minutes. Remove from the pan and place on a chopping board. Slice or shred.

Meanwhile heat the grill. Place the pitta strips on a baking tray and grill for 2–3 minutes until lightly toasted. Place the pepper and tomatoes on a separate baking tray. Grill for 5 minutes until softened and lightly golden. Remove from the oven and set aside.

Place the pepper and tomatoes in a bowl and add the onion, celery, olives, capers, cucumber, herbs.

Mix the oil, vinegar and garlic together. Drizzle over the salad and season to taste. Top with the sliced chicken and pitta strips.

Nutrition per serving: 398kcal, Fat 17g, of which saturates 2.9g, Carbohydrates 21g, of which sugars 11g, Fibre 5.7g, Protein 37g

LUNCH
Salads

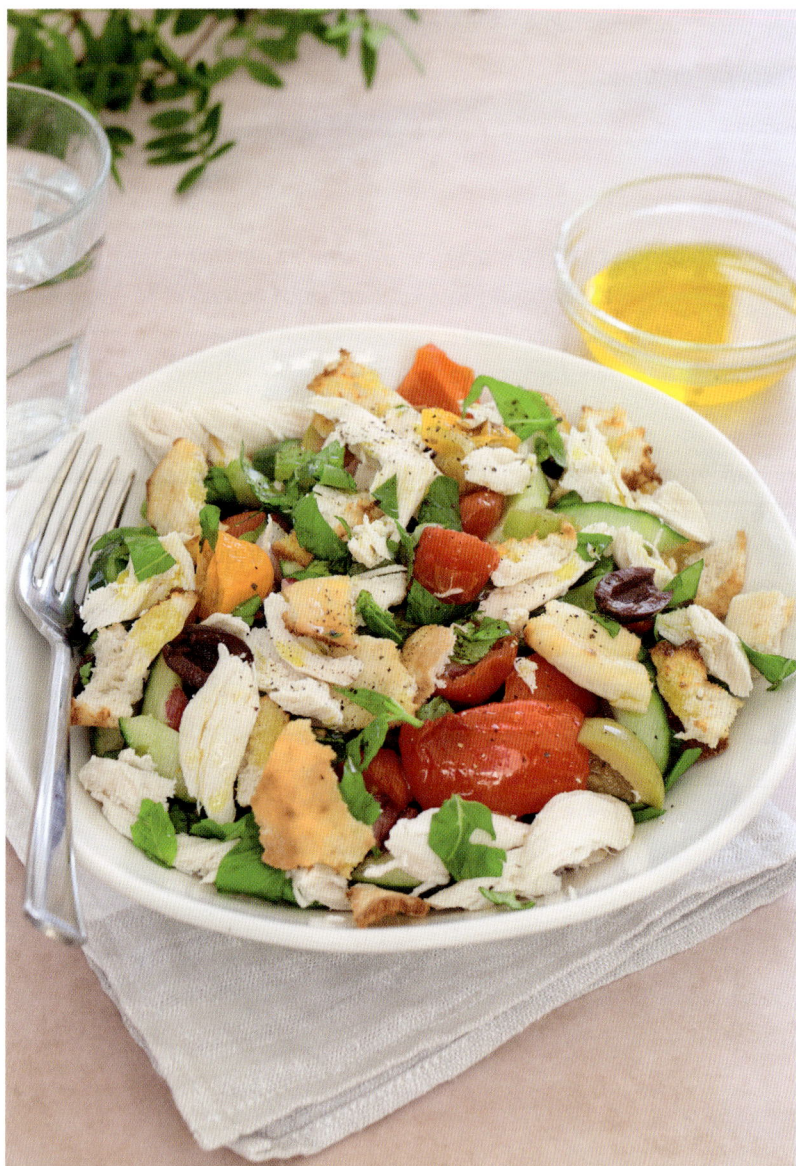

Prawn and Edamame Bean Salad

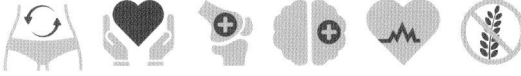

This vibrant, colourful Asian-style salad is packed with protein, omega-3 fatty acids and antioxidants. The array of vegetables and edamame beans provides plenty of fibre for a healthy gut and will help you feel fuller for longer.

Preparation time: 15 minutes

Cooking time: 3 minutes

Serves 2

Ingredients

- 2 tsp olive oil
- 200g raw prawns
- 1 carrot, julienne-cut
- ½ red pepper, deseeded and julienne-cut
- ½ cucumber, deseeded and thinly sliced

- 1 romaine lettuce, shredded
- 100g edamame beans, cooked
- ½ red chilli, deseeded and diced
- Handful of mint leaves, chopped
- Handful of coriander leaves, chopped
- 2 spring onions, finely chopped

Dressing

- 1 garlic clove, crushed
- ½ red chilli, deseeded and diced
- 1 tsp fresh ginger, peeled and chopped
- 1 tbsp fish sauce

- 2 tsp caster sugar
- Juice of 1 lime
- Black pepper
- 1 lemongrass stalk, lower part only chopped

Method

Make the dressing by placing everything in a blender and processing until smooth.

Heat the oil in a sauté pan and fry the prawns until pink and cooked, about 2–3 minutes. Remove from the pan and leave to cool.

Combine all the ingredients for the salad in a large bowl. Just before serving, add the dressing and toss well.

Nutrition per serving: 250kcal, Fat 8.5g, of which saturates 1g, Carbohydrates 14g, of which sugars 13g, Fibre 6.7g, Protein 25g

LUNCH
Salads

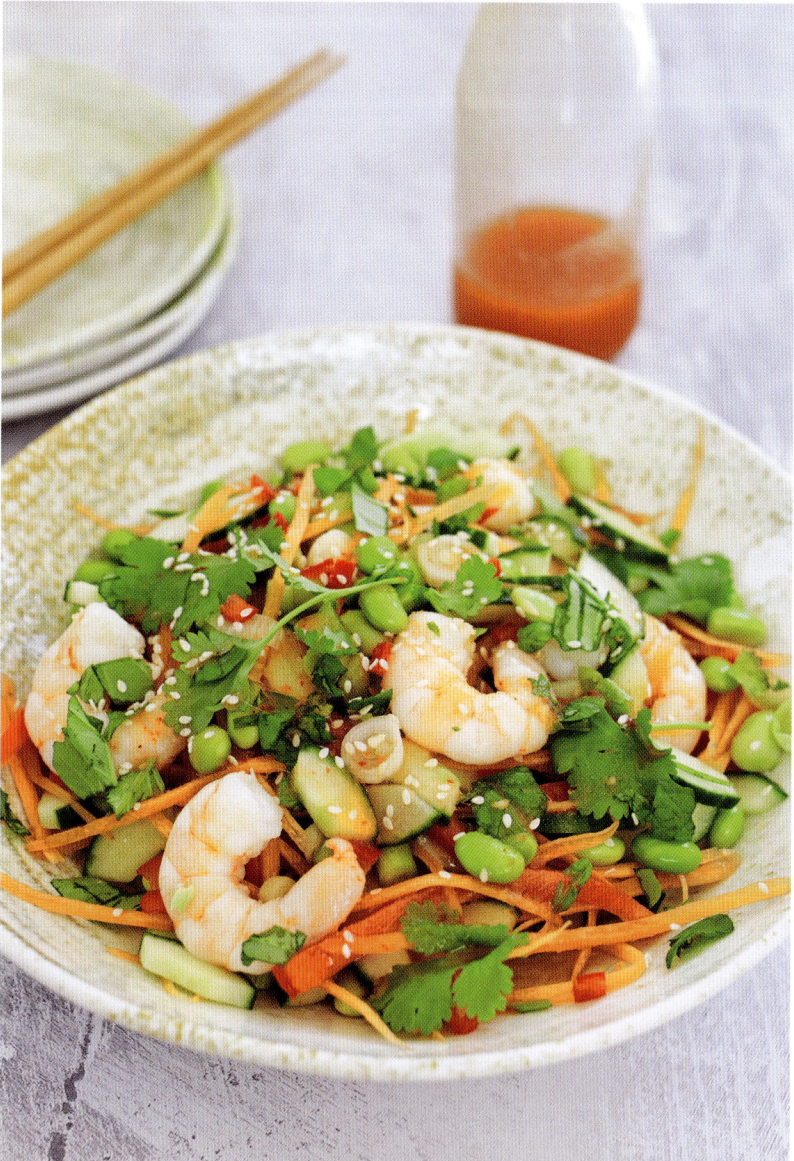

Mackerel, Roasted Beetroot and Potato Salad

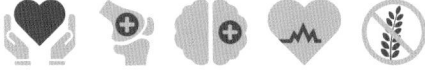

This is a simple, nutritious salad, combining the richness of mackerel with the earthy sweetness of beetroot. Mackerel is an excellent source of omega-3 fatty acids to help lower inflammation and support brain and heart health. Beetroot contains nitrates shown to improve blood circulation throughout the body.

Preparation time: 10 minutes

Cooking time: 25 minutes

Serves 2

Ingredients

- 4 raw small beetroot, cleaned (about 300g)
- 250g baby new potatoes, halved
- 2 tsp olive oil

Dressing

- 2 tsp natural yogurt
- 1 tsp lemon juice
- 2 tsp creamed horseradish sauce

To serve

- 2 smoked mackerel fillets, skinned and flaked
- 150g bag watercress or mixed leafy greens

Method

Preheat the oven to 200°C/Gas Mark 6.

Toss the beetroot and potatoes with the oil, season and roast for 20–25 minutes, until tender. Once cool, cut the beetroot into chunks.

Whisk together the yogurt, lemon juice and horseradish. Season to taste. Place the mackerel, watercress, beetroot and potatoes in a bowl. Drizzle over the dressing and lightly toss to serve.

Nutrition per serving: 514kcal, Fat 28g, of which saturates 5.9g, Carbohydrates 32g, of which sugars 15g, Fibre 7.9g, Protein 28g

LUNCH
Salads

MAINS
Meat

Slow-Roasted Lamb with Citrus Quinoa Salad

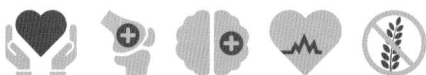

This slow-cooked lamb is simple to prepare and creates a wonderful melt-in-the-mouth meat, full of Middle Eastern flavours. Protein-rich, this is ideal for supporting muscle and bone health as well as immune function. The fruity quinoa salad is packed with protective antioxidants and plenty of fibre for blood sugar balance.

Preparation time: 20 minutes, plus marinating time

Cooking time: 5 hours, 15 minutes

Serves 4–6

Ingredients

- 2 onions
- 4 garlic cloves, crushed
- 2.5cm/1 inch fresh ginger root, peeled and chopped
- 1 tsp ground cinnamon
- 1 tsp ground cumin
- Pinch of turmeric

- 10g mint leaves, chopped
- Salt and black pepper
- 2 tbsp olive oil
- 1.5kg lamb shoulder, bone in
- 700ml chicken stock
- 1 tbsp apple cider vinegar

Salad

- 100g quinoa
- 200ml vegetable stock or water
- 2 large oranges
- 2 tsp sherry vinegar
- 2 tsp olive oil

- 60g pomegranate seeds
- 1 cucumber, deseeded and diced
- 4 tomatoes, deseeded and diced
- Handful of mint leaves, chopped
- Handful of parsley, chopped

Method

Roughly chop one of the onions. Put in a food processor with the garlic, ginger, spices and mint, and blitz with the oil and seasoning, to form a coarse paste. Add a little water if needed.

Pat dry the lamb and pierce the flesh all over using a small, sharp knife. Coat the lamb well with all the paste. Ideally place in the fridge for a few hours or overnight, to let the flavours develop.

Preheat the oven to 180°C/Gas Mark 4.

Cut the remaining onion into wedges and place in a large, deep roasting tin. Place the lamb on top and then pour the chicken stock and the apple cider vinegar around the lamb in the pan. Bake for 45 minutes, baste the lamb, and then cover the tin with foil and lower the heat to 140°C. Roast for 4 hours, occasionally basting the lamb with the stock as it cooks.

Turn the heat back up to 180°C/Gas Mark 4. Remove the foil and cook for 30 minutes until the lamb is well browned. Gently remove the lamb, place on a board and cover with foil. Drain the juices into a pan and simmer for a few minutes to reduce slightly, to make a sauce. Place the lamb on a deep platter and pour over the sauce.

While the lamb is cooking prepare the salad. Place the quinoa in a saucepan with the stock. Bring to the boil and then turn down to a gentle simmer. Cover and cook for 15 minutes. Turn off the heat and allow the quinoa to steam (lid on) for another 5 minutes.

To make the dressing, segment the oranges and set aside. Squeeze any residual juice from the pith into a small bowl, add the vinegar, oil and season. Place the quinoa in a bowl and mix in the orange segments, pomegranate seeds, cucumber, tomatoes and herbs. Drizzle over the dressing and toss lightly. Serve the lamb with the quinoa salad.

MAINS Meat

Nutrition per serving: 640kcal, Fat 44g, of which saturates 18g, Carbohydrates 19g, of which sugars 10g, Fibre 3.6g, Protein 40g

Moroccan Spiced Lamb Tagine

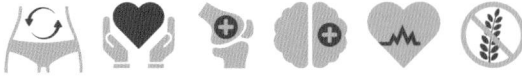

This fragrant, lightly spiced, one-pot stew takes little effort, making it ideal for busy days. You can even make it the day before and reheat it when ready to eat. Packed with an array of vegetables, it is nutrient-rich and packed with protein, to keep you energized throughout the day.

Preparation time: 15 minutes

Cooking time: 2 hours

Serves 4

Ingredients

- 2 tbsp olive oil
- 400g diced lamb
- 1 onion, finely chopped
- 2 garlic cloves, finely chopped
- 1 tsp ras el hanout
- ½ tsp ground coriander
- ½ tsp cinnamon
- ½ tsp ground cumin
- 300ml lamb or beef stock
- 1 x 400g can chopped tomatoes
- 2 courgettes, cut into chunks
- 200g butternut squash, diced
- 1 red pepper, cut into chunks
- 1 x 400g can chickpeas, drained and rinsed
- 2 tsp harissa paste
- Pinch of sea salt and black pepper, to taste
- 200g basmati rice (omit if on Reset)

To serve: Pomegranate seeds, flaked almonds and chopped parsley or mint

Method
Preheat the oven to 180°C/Gas Mark 4.

Heat the olive oil in a flameproof casserole dish over a high heat. Brown the lamb in batches and then set aside.

Add the onion and cook gently for 10 minutes, until soft and golden. Add the garlic and spices and cook for a further 2 minutes, then return the lamb to the casserole dish.

Add the stock and chopped tomatoes. Heat to simmering point, cover, and then cook in the oven for 1 hour. Add the courgette, butternut squash, red pepper, chickpeas, harissa and seasoning, and cook in the oven for a further 30 minutes. Meanwhile, cook the rice according to the packet instructions.

Once the tagine is cooked, scatter over pomegranate seeds, flaked almonds and chopped herbs. Serve the tagine over the cooked rice (omit rice if on Reset).

Nutrition per serving: 450kcal, Fat 15g, of which saturates 4.5g, Carbohydrates 49g, of which sugars 7.7g, Fibre 3.4g, Protein 27g

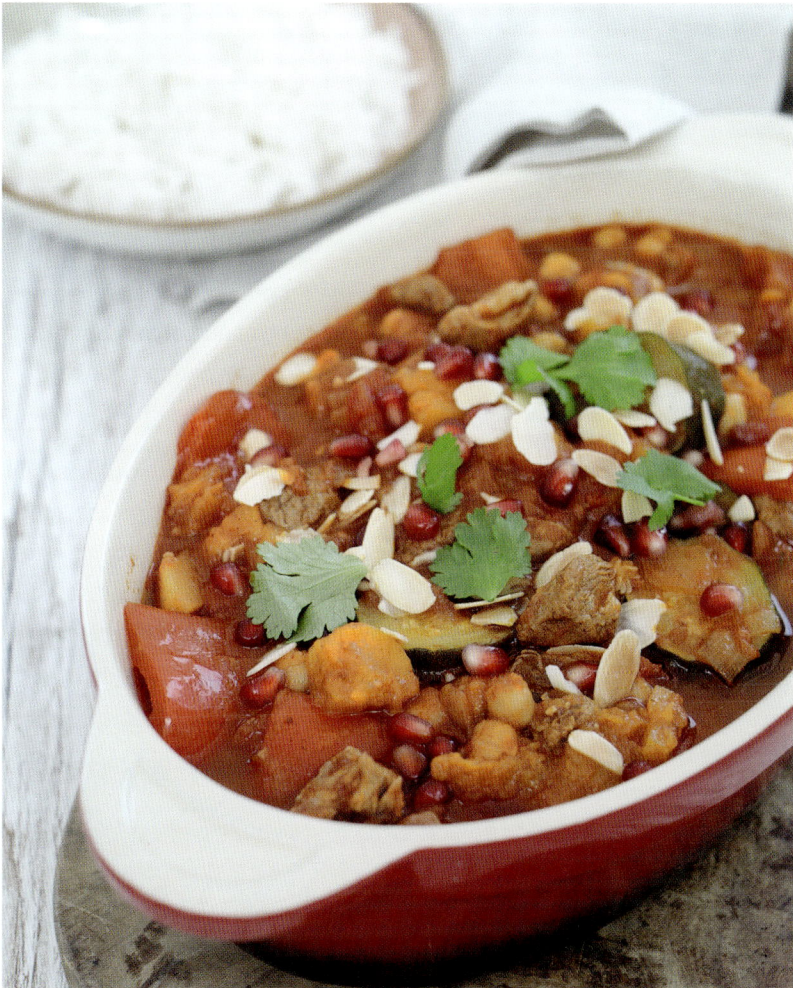

MAINS
Meat

One-Pan Beef and Lentil Chilli

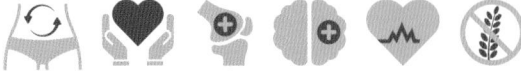

Delicious and simple to prepare, this one-pot meal is packed with protein, and adding beans and lentils is an easy way to sneak in more fibre and phyto-estrogens. It is perfect for an energy boost. You can also make this in a slow cooker (see instructions). Accompany with rice, if wished, or serve with tacos.

Preparation time: 10 minutes

Cooking time: 3 hours, 5 minutes

Serves 4

Ingredients

- 2 tsp olive oil
- 400g lean beef mince
- 1 onion, diced
- 1 red chilli, deseeded and diced
- 1 red pepper, deseeded and cut into chunks
- 2 tsp chipotle chilli flakes
- 1 tsp ground cumin
- 1 tsp ground coriander
- 2 tsp smoked paprika
- 2 garlic cloves, crushed
- 1 x 400g can green or brown lentils, drained and rinsed
- 1 x 400g can chopped tomatoes
- 1 x 400g can kidney beans, drained and rinsed
- 500ml beef stock
- Pinch of black pepper

To serve: 2 spring onions, chopped, Greek yogurt and mixed salad, rice or tacos (optional – omit if on Reset)

Method

Preheat the oven to 150°C/Gas Mark 3.

Heat the oil in a large ovenproof casserole dish. Add the beef mince and onion, and cook for 4–5 minutes, to brown the beef all over. Add all the remaining ingredients and stir well. Bring to a simmer, place the lid on the dish and put in the oven. Cook for 3 hours. If using a slow cooker you can cook on a low heat for 4–6 hours, or 3 hours on high heat.

MAINS
Meat

Top the chilli with spring onions and a spoonful of Greek yogurt. Accompany with a mixed salad.

> **Nutrition per serving:** 318kcal, Fat 7.8g of which saturates 2.7g, Carbohydrates 22g of which sugars 7.1g, Fibre 11g, Protein 33g

Baked Turkey Meatballs with Caponata

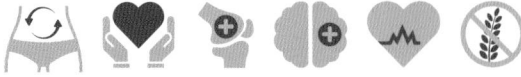

This is a wonderful Mediterranean-inspired dish. Caponata is a deliciously rich aubergine dish packed with antioxidants such as anthocyanins, which are known to have a protective effect for our cells. They also contain phyto-estrogens, which can have a mild oestrogen-like effect, making them particularly useful during the menopause transition. Turkey mince is lean and high in protein, B vitamins and choline – important for brain function. You can prepare the caponata the day before and reheat when ready to serve. The meatballs can also be air-fried.

Preparation time: 15 minutes

Cooking time: 40–60 minutes

Serves 4

Ingredients

- 450g lean turkey mince
- 1 egg
- 60g panko breadcrumbs (or dried gluten free breadcrumbs)
- 1 tbsp grated parmesan
- ½ tsp garlic salt
- ½ tsp dried thyme
- ½ tsp onion powder

Caponata

- 2 small aubergines, cut into cubes (about 400g)
- 2 tbsp olive oil
- ½ tsp sea salt and black pepper
- 1 small red onion, diced
- 2 garlic cloves, crushed
- 1 anchovy, chopped
- 2 x 400g cans chopped tomatoes
- 1 red pepper, cut into 1cm pieces
- 4 celery sticks, cut into 1cm pieces
- 60ml white wine vinegar
- 60ml red wine or stock
- 1 tbsp tomato puree
- 1 tbsp capers, drained
- 10 green olives, pitted
- 2 tsp sugar or maple syrup

To serve: Chopped parsley

Method

Heat the oven to 200°C/Gas Mark 6. Line 2 baking sheets with greaseproof paper and oil lightly.

To make the meatballs, simply place all the ingredients in a bowl and mix well together. Roll the mixture into around 28 balls. Place on the baking sheets and chill until ready to cook.

Meanwhile, make the caponata. Place the aubergine pieces on a baking tray and drizzle over 1 tbsp olive oil and season. Bake the aubergine for 20 minutes until golden and tender, and then remove from the oven.

Place the meatballs in the oven and bake for 20–25 minutes until golden and cooked through. Alternatively, air-fry in batches for 5–8 minutes until cooked.

Meanwhile, heat 1 tbsp olive oil in a large pan and sauté the onion, garlic and anchovy for a couple of minutes, and then add the chopped tomatoes and remaining ingredients, including the aubergine, and cook for 15 minutes covered, until the peppers and celery are soft and the mixture is thick. Toss in the meatballs and scatter with herbs to serve.

> **Nutrition per serving:** 328kcal, Fat 12g, of which saturates 2.8g, Carbohydrates 27g, of which sugars 16g, Fibre 6g, Protein 24g

MAINS
Meat

Smoky Chipotle Chicken with Chunky Guacamole

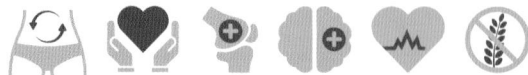

This is a simple Mexican one-pot meal that is rich in protein to support muscle mass, stave off hunger and balance blood sugar levels. Avocados are a great source of healthy fats, fibre, potassium and folate, making them particularly beneficial for heart health.

Preparation time: 15 minutes

Cooking time: 50 minutes

Serves 2

Ingredients

- 1 tbsp olive oil
- 2 chicken thigh fillets, boneless, halved
- ½ red onion, cut into wedges
- 1 red pepper, deseeded and cut into chunks
- 1 garlic clove, crushed
- ½ tsp ground cumin
- 1 tsp smoked paprika

- 2 tsp chipotle chilli paste
- 1 x 400g can chopped tomatoes
- 1 x 400g can black beans or kidney beans, drained and rinsed
- 100ml water or chicken stock
- ½ tsp cocoa powder
- 1 x 198g can sweetcorn, drained
- Handful of coriander leaves
- Salt and pepper

For the guacamole

- ½ ripe avocado
- Salt to taste
- Drizzle of extra virgin olive oil
- Juice of ½ lime (or to taste)

- 1 spring onion, chopped
- 1 tbsp fresh coriander leaves, chopped

To serve: Mixed salad and a small handful of tortilla chips (optional)

Method

Preheat the oven to 180°C/Gas Mark 4.

MAINS
Meat

Heat the oil in a large ovenproof casserole dish. Season the chicken thigh fillets and brown them all over on a high heat, for 2–3 minutes. Remove from the pan and place on a plate.

Add the onion and pepper to the pan and sauté gently for 2 minutes, then add the garlic and spices and stir for a minute to enhance the flavour.

Return the chicken to the casserole dish and stir to coat in the spices. Add the tomatoes and black beans, stock, cocoa powder and season. Bring to a simmer, cover and transfer to the oven to cook for 45 minutes, until the chicken is tender. Remove from the heat, stir in the sweetcorn and sprinkle over the coriander.

Meanwhile, make the guacamole. Chop the avocado and place in a bowl with the remaining ingredients, and mash lightly to create a coarse texture. Season to taste.

Serve the chipotle chicken alongside the guacamole, tortilla chips and a mixed salad.

Nutrition per serving: 576kcal, Fat 24g, of which saturates 5.1g, Carbohydrates 42g, of which sugars 26g, Fibre 19g, Protein 37g

MAINS
Meat

Thai Green Chicken Curry

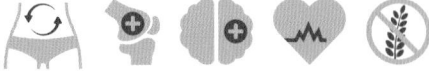

This creamy curry is packed with anti-inflammatory herbs and spices. Wonderfully green and vibrant, it is crammed with plenty of nutrient-rich vegetables. You could replace the chicken with pan-fried tofu or tempeh, if wished.

Preparation time: 15 minutes

Cooking time: 25 minutes

Serves 2

Ingredients
Thai green curry sauce

- 1 spring onion, chopped
- ½ green chilli, deseeded and chopped
- 1 stick lemongrass, finely chopped
- 1 garlic clove, crushed
- 1 tsp fresh ginger, crushed
- Handful of coriander leaves
- 1 tbsp tamari soy sauce
- 2 tsp rice vinegar
- 1 tsp maple syrup
- ½ tsp turmeric
- 1 x 300ml can light coconut milk
- Pinch of salt

Curry

- 2 tsp olive oil
- 2 chicken breasts, cut into chunks (or 250g tofu or tempeh)
- 50g asparagus, trimmed and halved (or green beans)
- 50g sugar snap peas or mangetout
- 100g broccoli, cut into small florets
- 60g frozen peas, thawed
- Large handful of baby spinach

To serve: 100g basmati rice, rinsed (omit if on Reset), sesame seeds to sprinkle, 1 tsp chopped mint leaves and lime wedges (optional)

Method

To make the Thai green curry sauce, place everything in a high-speed blender and process until smooth.

Put the rice in a pan and add 200ml water. Bring to the boil, cover with a lid and lower the heat to a very gentle simmer. Cook for 20 minutes and then turn off the heat without removing the lid, and allow it to steam for a further 5 minutes.

While the rice is cooking, make the curry. Heat the oil in a large sauté pan and pan-fry the chicken until white and lightly golden all over – about 5 minutes. If using tofu or tempeh, cut into bite-size cubes and pan-fry in a little oil before adding to the curry Add asparagus, sugar snap peas and broccoli and continue to cook, stirring for another 3–4 minutes, until the vegetables are lightly cooked but still crisp.

Add the curry sauce and bring to a simmer, then cover and simmer for about 10 minutes, until the chicken is cooked through and vegetables are just tender. Add the peas and spinach and cook for a further 3–4 minutes.

Serve with the cooked rice and top with sesame seeds and fresh mint leaves. Accompany with lime wedges.

Nutrition per serving: 436kcal, Fat 9.3g, of which saturates 6.7g, Carbohydrates 49g, of which sugars 6.9g, Fibre 6.1g, Protein 36g

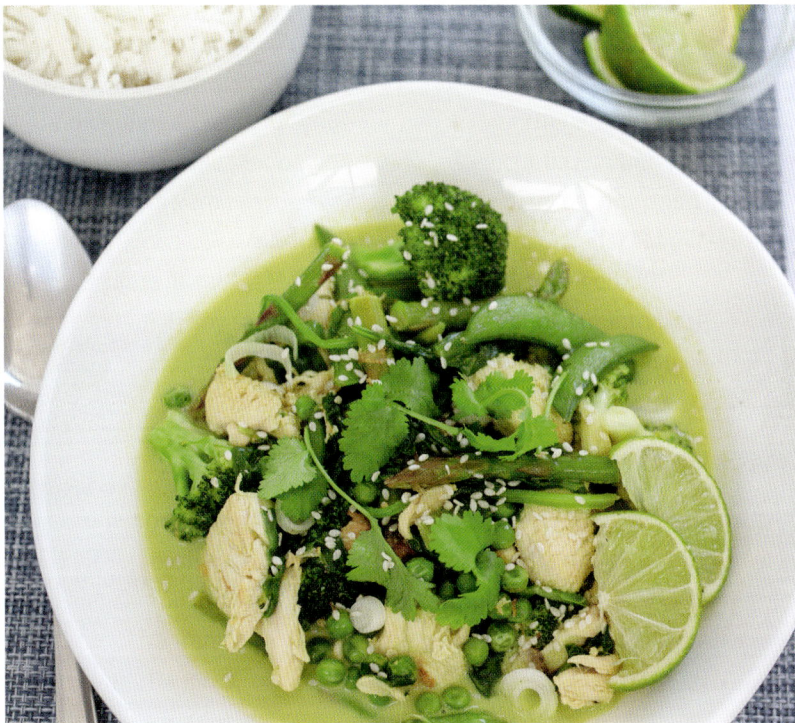

MAINS
Meat

Pomegranate-Griddled Chicken with Aubergine

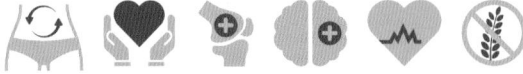

Sweet and sticky pomegranate molasses is a wonderful marinade for chicken and fish. Pomegranates are rich in vitamin C, carotenoids and anthocyanidins, as well as protective antioxidants that are beneficial for the heart and skin health. This is a high-protein dish, ideal for keeping hunger pangs at bay.

Preparation time: 15 minutes, plus marinating time

Cooking time: 35 minutes

Serves 2

Ingredients

- 2 chicken breasts, skinless (250g)
- 1 tbsp pomegranate molasses
- ½ tsp cinnamon
- 2 garlic cloves, crushed
- 1 tsp olive oil
- 1 aubergine, cut into chunks
- Salt and pepper

Salad

- 150g green beans, trimmed and halved
- 100g bag mixed salad leaves
- 8 cherry tomatoes, halved
- ½ red onion, finely chopped
- 30g pomegranate seeds
- Handful of parsley, chopped

Dressing

- 3 tbsp pomegranate molasses
- 2 tbsp lemon juice
- Pinch of ground cumin
- ½ tsp caster sugar
- 2 tbsp olive oil
- Salt and pepper
- A little water to thin

Method

Place the chicken breasts between sheets of cling film and bash gently to flatten out.

Combine the pomegranate molasses, cinnamon, garlic and oil, and season. Rub the mixture all over the chicken breast and leave to marinate for at least 30 minutes in the fridge.

Whisk all the ingredients for the dressing and set aside.

Meanwhile, cut the aubergine into small chunks. Place in a roasting tin and toss through 1 tbsp of the dressing.

Preheat the oven to 200°C/Gas Mark 6. Roast the aubergine for 18–20 minutes, until golden. Stir occasionally.

Cook the green beans in a pan of boiling water for 3–4 minutes until just tender, then drain well.

Heat a griddle pan. Griddle the chicken breasts in batches on each side (4–5 minutes) until cooked through. Alternatively, place under a grill and grill on each side for 6–8 minutes, until cooked.

Mix the salad leaves with the cherry tomatoes, red onion, green beans, pomegranate seeds and parsley. Scatter over the aubergine. Drizzle over the dressing and serve with the chicken.

Nutrition per serving: 457kcal, Fat 17g, of which saturates 2.7g, Carbohydrates 35g, of which sugars 33g, Fibre 6.8g, Protein 34g

MAINS
Meat

MAINS
Fish

Indonesian Fish Curry

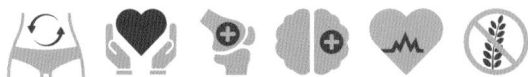

This fish curry uses cod, which is high in protein and a good source of iodine, an important mineral for thyroid function. It also provides B vitamins for energy, brain and heart health. This curry is served with cauliflower rice, which is packed with vitamins C and K, B vitamins, and choline, which is important for liver function and brain health. This is an ideal dish for Reset days, and being high in fibre will help reduce hunger pangs.

Preparation time: 15 minutes

Cooking time: 18 minutes

Serves 2

Ingredients

- 250g cod fillet, boneless, skinless
- 2 tsp olive oil
- ½ onion, finely chopped
- 1 red pepper, cut into chunks
- 2cm/1 inch piece fresh ginger, peeled and finely grated
- 2 garlic cloves, crushed
- 1 tsp ground coriander
- 1 tsp ground cumin
- ½ tsp turmeric
- Pinch of chilli flakes
- 1 tbsp tamari soy sauce
- 1 tsp lemongrass paste
- 1 tsp tamarind (optional)
- 1 x 400ml can light coconut milk
- 200g green beans, trimmed
- 100g baby spinach leaves

Cauliflower rice

- ½ cauliflower
- 2 tsp olive oil
- Salt and pepper to taste
- Handful of coriander leaves

To serve: Lime wedges and 1 tbsp cashew nuts, toasted

Method

Cut the cod into 4cm chunks and set aside.

Heat the oil in a large, deep sauté pan over a medium-low heat. When hot, add the onion and pepper, and fry gently for 5 minutes, or until softened. Add the ginger, garlic and spices, tamari, lemongrass paste, tamarind and coconut milk. Simmer for 5 minutes. Add the green beans and simmer for a further 5 minutes, to reduce the liquid. Stir in the spinach to wilt down.

Add the pieces of cod to the pan and simmer gently for 2–3 minutes, being careful not to break the fish up. The fish will turn opaque when cooked and the spinach will have wilted.

To make the cauliflower rice place the florets into a food processor in batches and pulse briefly until broken into small bits resembling rice. Alternatively, you can use a box grater. Place the cauliflower in a clean tea towel and lightly press to remove excess moisture. Heat the oil in a frying pan and add the cauliflower rice, salt and a little pepper. Cook, stirring occasionally, until the cauliflower is crisp and tender and starts to turn a light brown – about 6 minutes. Stir through the coriander leaves.

Serve the curry over the cauliflower rice with lime wedges if wished. Scatter over the cashew nuts to serve.

> **Nutrition per serving:** 455kcal, Fat 26g, of which saturates 14g, Carbohydrates 21g, of which sugars 12g, Fibre 8.6g, Protein 32g

MAINS
Fish

Fish Tacos with Pickled Red Onions

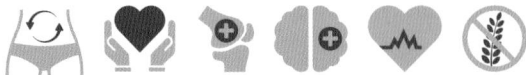

Packed with flavour, this is a great way to include more fish in your diet. With just a handful of ingredients, this is perfect for busy days. The pickled onions can be kept in the fridge for 3–4 days and are delicious added to salads.

Preparation time: 10 minutes

Marinating time: 20 minutes

Cooking time: 13 minutes

Serves 2

Ingredients

- 325g cod, pollock or haddock fillets, skinned
- 1 tbsp chipotle paste
- ½ tsp ground cumin
- ½ tsp smoked paprika
- Juice of 1 lime
- 1 tsp olive oil
- Pinch of salt

Pickled onions

- 1 red onion, very thinly sliced
- 1 lime, juice only
- 1 tbsp apple cider vinegar
- Pinch of sea salt
- Pinch of sugar

To serve: Shredded lettuce, sliced avocado (optional), 4 small corn or wheat tortilla wraps and salsa (optional)

Method

Prepare the pickled onions. Mix the very thinly sliced red onion with the lime juice, vinegar and a pinch of salt and sugar, and set aside for at least 20 minutes (this can be prepared a day ahead).

Combine the chipotle paste, cumin, paprika, lime juice and oil with a little salt in a large bowl. Toss the fish fillets in the spiced lime paste and set aside for 10–15 minutes, to allow the flavours to develop.

Heat the grill to high. Line a baking tray with foil and brush with a little oil, place the fish fillets on the tray, pour over any leftover paste from the bowl and brush with a little more oil. Cook the fish for around 6–7 mins until cooked through and starting to scorch in places. Remove from the oven and break into large chunks.

Warm the wraps in the oven for a couple of minutes or microwave briefly. To serve, place the lettuce on the warm wraps, spoon on the fish, and then top with some sliced avocado, pickled onions and salsa, if using.

Nutrition per serving: 354kcal, Fat 12g, of which saturates 2.4, Carbohydrates 26g, of which sugars 4.4g, Fibre 2.1g, Protein 31g

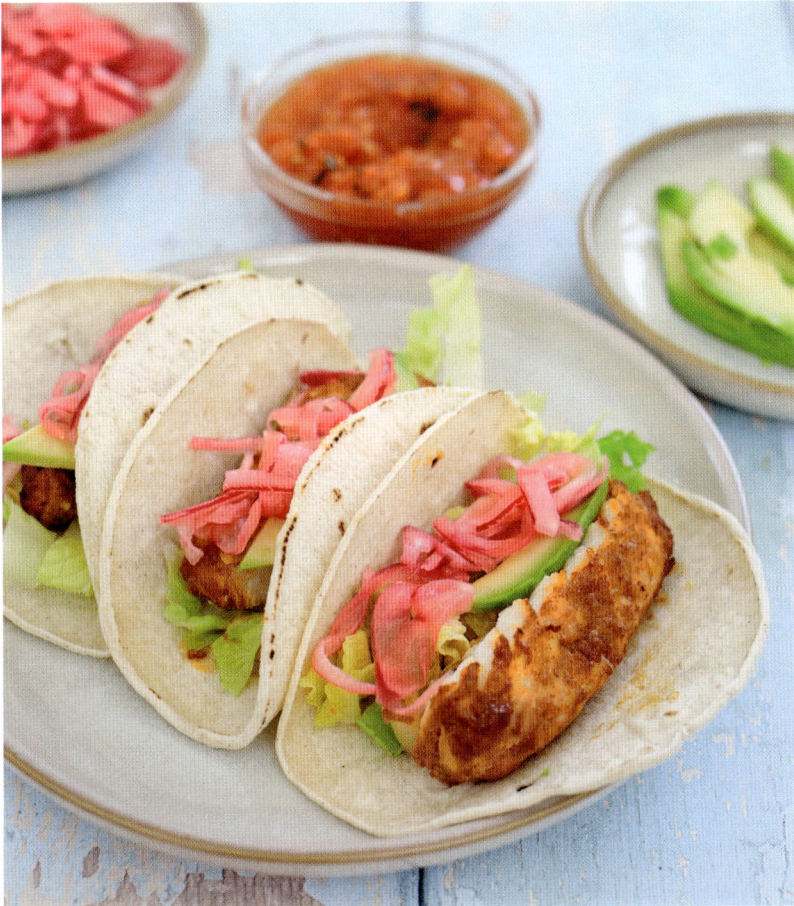

MAINS
Fish

Baked Sea Bass with Gremolata and Fennel Salad

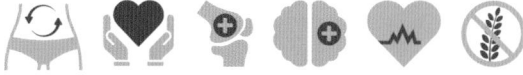

Sea bass is rich in omega-3 fatty acids and vitamin D, which is important for heart, bone and brain health. The herby salad is packed with antioxidants and vitamin C for collagen synthesis and protecting cells from free radical damage. You could prepare the salad the day before if wished.

Preparation time: 20 minutes

Cooking time: 6 minutes

Serves 2

Ingredients

- 2 sea bass fillets, boneless (300g)
- 1 tbsp olive oil
- Sea salt and black pepper

Gremolata

- 15g parsley, finely chopped
- 1 clove garlic, finely crushed
- Zest and juice ½ lemon
- Sea salt and black pepper

Fennel salad

- 4 mint leaves, roughly chopped
- Small handful of dill, chopped
- Small handful of chives, chopped
- 1 tbsp olive oil
- Salt and pepper
- 1 preserved lemon, flesh and pips removed and skin chopped
- 1 tbsp lemon juice
- 1 fennel bulb, trimmed, halved lengthways and finely shaved (on a mandolin, knife or shredder in the food processor)
- 1 courgette, finely shaved lengthways (using a swivel potato peeler)
- Pinch of fennel seeds

Method

To make the gremolata, mix together the parsley, garlic, lemon zest and juice, and season with salt and pepper.

To make the fennel salad, put the herbs, oil and a pinch of salt and pepper, preserved lemon and lemon juice in the food processor and blitz to combine. Place the fennel and courgette in a bowl with the fennel seeds, salt and pepper. Pour over the herb mixture and toss well.

Season the fish with salt and pepper. Heat the oil in a frying pan over a medium-high heat, then add the fish, skin-side down, and fry for 3–4 minutes, until the skin is golden and the fish is almost cooked. Turn and cook the other side for 1–2 minutes, depending on the thickness of the fillet.

Pile the salad on to plates and top with the sea bass. Drizzle over a little gremolata to serve.

> **Nutrition per serving:** 399kcal, Fat 28g of which saturates 5.1g, Carbohydrates 2.9g, of which sugars 2.4g, Fibre 2.9g, Protein 32g

MAINS
Fish

Roasted Oriental Trout

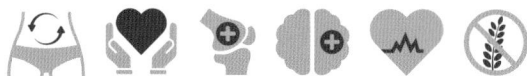

Trout are an excellent source of protein, B vitamins and omega-3 fatty acids to support brain and heart health. Omega-3 helps lower inflammation and may be useful for issues such as joint pain and hot flushes. Salmon can be used instead of trout. This is delicious served hot or cold with salad or stir-fry vegetables.

Preparation time: 10 minutes, plus marinating time

Cooking time: 25 minutes

Serves 2

Ingredients

- 2 small trout, cleaned and scaled, or 1 boneless salmon side (about 400g)

Marinade

- 50ml tamari soy sauce
- 50ml rice wine vinegar
- 2 garlic cloves, crushed
- 1 spring onion, finely chopped
- 2cm/1 inch piece of fresh root ginger, grated
- 2 tbsp honey or maple syrup
- 2 star anise

To serve: Fresh coriander leaves and lime wedges

Method

Clean the trout or salmon under cold running water. If using trout, make several diagonal slashes on either side of the fish and then place in a large dish. To make the marinade, mix all the ingredients together. Coat the fish with the marinade, cover and chill for 2 hours.

Place the fish on a large piece of foil (large enough to enclose the fish) and spoon over some of the marinade. Loosely cover the fish with the foil to make a parcel, leaving space in the parcel for air to circulate around the fish.

Place on a baking tray and cook in a preheated oven at 200°C/Gas Mark 6 for 20 minutes, or until the fish is cooked through.

Open the foil parcel and then grill for 2–3 minutes to crisp up the skin. You can place any remaining marinade in a small pan and simmer until syrupy, then spoon over the fish.

Garnish with fresh coriander leaves and lime wedges.

Nutrition per serving: 352kcal, Fat 11g, of which saturates 2.4g, Carbohydrates 18g, of which sugars 16g, Fibre 0.5g, Protein 43g

MAINS
Fish

Smoked Salmon and Herb Fish Cakes

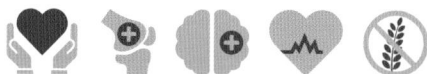

These are flaky, golden fish cakes that are full of flavour with the addition of smoked salmon, mackerel and herbs. They are a great source of omega-3 fatty acids, vitamin D, B vitamins and magnesium, making them beneficial for brain, heart and bone health. The tartare-style source provides probiotics to support gut health. You can make up a big batch of these fish cakes and freeze them cooked, ready to warm up when needed.

Preparation time: 15 minutes

Cooking time: 30 minutes

Makes 6

Ingredients

- 400g potatoes, peeled and cut into chunks
- 100g smoked salmon, cut into chunks
- 100g smoked mackerel, skinned and flaked
- 1 tbsp chopped dill
- 1 tbsp chopped parsley
- 2 tbsp horseradish sauce or yogurt
- 1 spring onion, chopped
- 1 tsp capers, rinsed and roughly chopped
- Zest of 1 lemon
- Sea salt and black pepper

Coating

- 1 egg, beaten
- 20g plain flour (or gluten-free flour)
- 60g dried breadcrumbs (or gluten-free dried breadcrumbs)
- Oil for frying

Tartare-style sauce

- 6 tbsp natural yogurt
- 1 tbsp capers, chopped
- 2 tbsp gherkins, chopped
- 1 garlic clove, crushed (optional)
- Zest and juice of ½ lemon

Method

Boil the potatoes in salted water for 5–7 minutes until tender, drain them well and then roughly mash them (they don't have to be smooth). Place the mash in a bowl, add the salmon and flake in the mackerel. Add the herbs, horseradish, spring onion, capers and lemon zest, setting aside a little zest to garnish, then season with salt and pepper. Mix everything together, taking care not to break up the mackerel too much. Using your hands, shape into six fish cakes.

Place the egg, flour, and breadcrumbs in three separate bowls. Season the flour with salt and pepper and dip the fish cakes first into the flour, then the egg, and finish off in the breadcrumbs.

Heat the oil in the pan and cook the fish cakes for 5 minutes on each side. If you wish, finish them off in the oven at 200°C/Gas Mark 6 for 10 minutes, to ensure even browning all over.

Mix together all the ingredients for the tartare-style sauce. Serve with the fish cakes and accompany with salad.

Nutrition per 2 fishcakes: 437kcal, Fat 15g, of which saturates 3.9g, Carbohydrates 48g, of which sugars 6.8g, Fibre 4.3g, Protein 25g

MAINS
Fish

Traybake Salmon with Pak Choi and Tomatoes

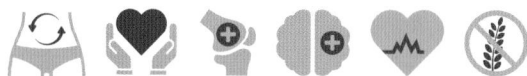

This easy, flavourful dish is perfect for a quick worknight dinner. Baked in one roasting tin, it is a simple dish to throw together. Simply accompany with a mixed salad for a high-protein meal. Salmon is an excellent source of omega-3 fatty acids, which can help boost mood and support bone health by lowering inflammation.

Preparation time: 10 minutes

Cooking time: 20 minutes

Serves 2

Marinade

- 3 tbsp tamari soy sauce
- 1 tsp brown sugar
- ½ tsp sesame oil
- 2cm ginger, finely grated
- 1 tsp fish sauce (optional)
- 4 baby pak choi, halved lengthwise (200g)
- 2 salmon fillets (300g)
- 100g cherry tomatoes, halved

To serve: ½ red chilli, thinly sliced, handful of chopped coriander leaves

Method

Preheat the oven to 180°C/Gas Mark 4. Line a baking tray with baking paper.

Combine the tamari soy sauce, sugar, oil, ginger and fish sauce in a large bowl. Place the pak choi on the baking tray and top with the salmon. Pour over the dressing.

Cover the tray with foil and bake in the oven for 15 minutes. Remove the foil, then scatter over the cherry tomatoes. Place back in the oven for a further 5 minutes, to soften the tomatoes.

Scatter with coriander leaves and chilli before serving.

Nutrition per serving: 395kcal, Fat 24g, of which saturates 4.5g, Carbohydrates 6.8g, of which sugars 5.5g, Fibre 3.2g, Protein 35g

MAINS
Vegetarian and Vegan

Black Bean Veggie Burgers

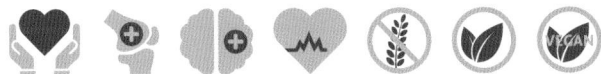

These chunky burgers, packed with a smoky flavour, are a great source of protein and fibre to help keep blood sugar balanced. Black beans are rich in antioxidants, particularly flavonoids, which can help reduce oxidative damage in the body and support heart health. Rich in B vitamins, they make an delicious, energizing dish.

Preparation time: 15 minutes

Cooking time: 15 minutes

Makes 6 burgers

Ingredients

- 1 tbsp olive oil
- 1 red onion, finely chopped
- 1 carrot, grated
- 1 garlic clove, crushed
- 120g chestnut or portobello mushrooms, finely chopped
- 1 x 400g can black beans or kidney beans, drained
- 2 tbsp tamari soy sauce
- 1 tbsp smoked paprika
- Pinch of chilli powder
- 4 tbsp porridge oats (or gluten-free oats)
- 2 tbsp nutritional yeast flakes

Method

Heat the olive oil in a medium frying pan, then sauté the onion, carrot, garlic and mushrooms for 3–5 minutes, to soften.

Place the beans in a food processor with the mushroom mixture and the rest of the ingredients and pulse to combine. You want a little texture, so do not blitz it for long. Divide the mixture into six portions and, using your hands, mould each portion into a burger shape.

You can either fry the burgers in a little olive oil for 5 minutes on each side or bake in the oven (200°C/Gas Mark 6) for 20 minutes, until golden.

Nutrition per burger: 120kcal, Fat 3.3g, of which saturates 0.5g, Carbohydrates 13g, of which sugars 4.4g, Fibre 5.8g, Protein 7.1g

Pulled Jackfruit Rolls

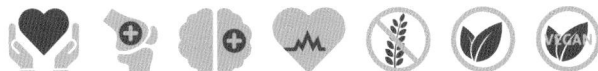

Lightly spiced with a rich, smoky, tomato sauce, these pulled jackfruit rolls are the perfect plant-based lunch or light meal. To really develop the flavour, make the mixture a day ahead and then reheat when ready to eat them. You can serve them in tacos instead of rolls, if wished. Jackfruit is rich in vitamin C, which is required for collagen production – important for skin, bones and joints. Jackfruit is also a useful source of fibre to help support digestive health and keep you feeling fuller for longer.

Preparation time: 10 minutes

Cooking time: 16 minutes

Serves 2

Ingredients

- 1 x 400g can jackfruit, drained and rinsed
- 2 tsp olive oil
- ½ red onion, diced
- 1 clove garlic, crushed
- 1 tsp smoked paprika
- ½ tsp ground cumin
- ½ tsp ground coriander
- Pinch of chilli powder or cayenne pepper
- Salt and black pepper
- 1 tbsp tamari soy sauce
- 200g passata
- 2 tsp honey or maple syrup
- 2 tsp apple cider vinegar

To serve: 2 seeded rolls, pickled onions (see Fish Tacos with Picked Red Onions on page 196), lettuce, mayonnaise or vegan mayonnaise

Method

Remove any tough parts from the jackfruit. With a fork, break it up into shreds.

Heat the oil in a frying pan and sauté the onion and garlic for 2–3 minutes. Add the spices and stir to coat in the oil. Add the jackfruit and mix thoroughly. Sauté for 2–3 minutes.

MAINS
Vegetarian and Vegan

Add the remaining ingredients to the frying pan and stir. Simmer for 10 minutes to reduce the liquid and let the flavours develop.

Serve in rolls with lettuce, picked onions and mayonnaise.

Nutrition per serving with a roll: 324kcal, Fat 6g, of which saturates 0.9g, Carbohydrates 51g, of which sugars 12g, Fibre 11g, Protein 9.1g

Mushroom Shawarma with Tahini Yogurt

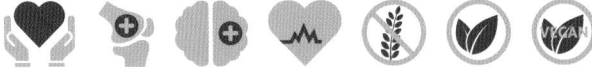

Shredded oyster mushrooms are marinated in a Middle Eastern-style sauce before pan frying, to create a delicious vegan 'shawarma'-style dish served with tahini yogurt. Tahini is a good source of calcium and magnesium to support bone health, while the yogurt supports gut and immune health. Oyster mushrooms, like other mushrooms, are rich in fibre, including beta glucans, which are known to support immune and heart health.

Preparation time: 20 minutes

Marinating time: 20–30 minutes

Cooking time: 6 minutes

Serves 2

Ingredients

- 300g oyster mushrooms

Marinade

- Juice of 1 orange
- 3 tbsp tamari soy sauce
- 1 tsp sumac
- Pinch of chilli powder
- Handful of coriander, chopped
- 1 tsp ground cumin
- 1 tsp smoked paprika
- 2 tsp olive oil
- Juice of ½ lime
- Black pepper

Salad

- ¼ cucumber, deseeded and diced
- ¼ red onion, diced
- 1 tomato, deseeded and diced
- 120g (or ½ can) chickpeas, drained and rinsed (or use toasted chickpeas – see Salt and Vinegar Roasted Chickpeas on page 226)
- 1 roasted red pepper, chopped
- 1 romaine lettuce, shredded
- Handful of parsley, chopped
- 1 tbsp lemon juice
- 2 tsp olive oil
- Salt and pepper to taste

MAINS
Vegetarian and Vegan

Tahini yogurt

- 1 tbsp runny tahini
- 3 tbsp low-fat natural yoghurt (or soy yogurt)
- ½ clove garlic, crushed
- 1 tbsp lemon juice
- Salt and pepper

To serve: 2 pitta breads or flatbreads

Method

Tear the mushrooms to form thick shreds. Place in a bowl and add all the ingredients for the marinade. Mix well and chill for at least 20–30 minutes. Tip the mushrooms and the marinade into a frying pan and sauté for about 5–6 minutes, until most of the liquid has evaporated.

Meanwhile, make up the salad. Simply toss the cucumber, onion, tomato, chickpeas, pepper, lettuce and parsley together in a bowl. Mix the lemon juice and olive oil together and season. Drizzle over the salad and toss well.

Make up the tahini yogurt by whisking all the ingredient together. Spread a little of the tahini yogurt over warmed flatbreads or a pitta and top with the mushrooms. Serve with the salad.

> **Nutrition per serving (with a pitta):** 548kcal, Fat 18g, of which saturates 2.9g, Carbohydrates 68g, of which sugars 19g, Fibre 15g, Protein 22g

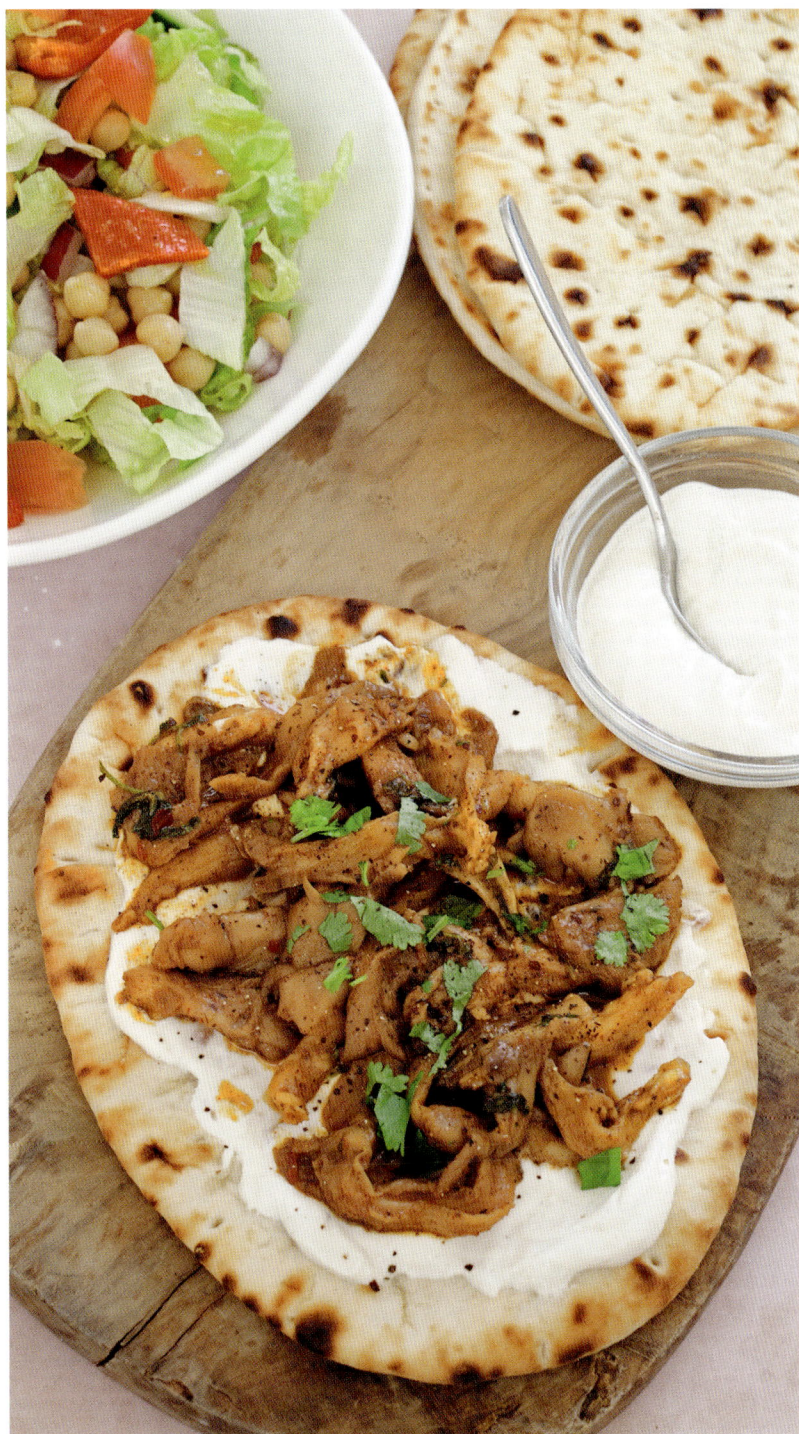

Chickpea Meatballs with BBQ Sauce

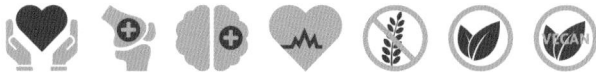

Quick and easy, these chickpea meatballs are loaded with flavour and served with a rich, smoky BBQ sauce. The chickpea meatballs can be air-fried. You can prepare the sauce ahead and reheat when needed. This is a low-carb meal, ideal for Reset days. High in fibre, chickpeas can help with digestion and bowel regularity. They are also a good source of phytoestrogens, which can have a mild oestrogen effect.

Preparation time: 15 minutes

Cooking time: 18 minutes

Serves 2

Ingredients

- 1 x 400g can chickpeas, drained
- ½ red onion
- 2 tsp taco spice mix
- 1 tsp smoked paprika
- 1 tbsp nutritional yeast flakes
- 1 egg
- Salt and pepper
- 80g dried breadcrumbs (or gluten-free dried breadcrumbs)
- 2 tsp olive oil

BBQ sauce

- ½ red onion, chopped
- 1 garlic clove, crushed
- ½ tsp Dijon mustard
- 1 tbsp maple syrup or honey
- 60g sundried tomatoes in oil, drained
- 1 x 400g can chopped tomatoes
- 2 tbsp apple cider vinegar
- 2 tbsp tamari soy sauce
- ½ tsp smoked paprika
- Pinch of chilli flakes
- Sea salt and black pepper

Method

Place all the ingredients for the chickpea meatballs (except the breadcrumbs) in a food processor and blitz to create a thick, slightly chunky paste. Spoon into a bowl and add half the breadcrumbs. Stir well. Take small pieces of the mixture and roll into walnut-size balls. Tip the remaining breadcrumbs on a tray and roll the chickpea balls in the breadcrumbs.

Heat the oil in a large frying pan over a medium heat. Once hot, add the chickpea meatballs in batches and cook for 6–8 minutes, turning to brown all sides, until golden. Alternatively, preheat an air fryer and cook in batches for around 8–10 minutes, until golden.

While the chickpea meatballs are cooking, make the BBQ sauce. Place all the ingredients in a blender or food processor and process until smooth. Pour into a pan and simmer gently for 6–8 minutes. Toss in the chickpea meatballs and serve.

Nutrition per serving: 503kcal, Fat 12g, of which saturates 2g, Carbohydrates 62g, of which sugars 26g, Fibre 14g, Protein 23g

Tofu Vegetable Medley

This is an easy recipe that can be batch-cooked and frozen if wished. You can pan-fry or air-fry the tofu. Instead of tofu, you can use 200g tempeh or 200g chicken breasts.

Preparation time: 15 minutes

Cooking time: 20 minutes

Serves 2

Ingredients

- 300g firm tofu, bite-size cubes
- 2 tsp olive oil
- 200g shiitake mushrooms, sliced
- 100g spinach
- 200g green beans, sliced in half
- 1 red pepper, cut into chunks
- Salt and pepper to taste

Marinade

- 2 tbsp soy sauce (or gluten-free soy sauce)
- Juice and zest of 1 lime
- 1 tsp fresh ginger, grated
- Drizzle of sriracha (to taste)

Method

Place the tofu in a bowl. Drizzle over the marinade of soy sauce, lime juice, ginger and sriracha, and toss well. Leave to marinate for at least 5 minutes. Air-fry the tofu for 5 minutes until golden (reserving the marinade) or add the tofu to a sauté pan with the marinade and cook for 6–7 minutes until lightly golden. Remove the tofu from the pan. Add the oil to the pan and sauté the vegetables over a low-medium heat for 10 minutes, stirring throughout. Season with salt and pepper.

Add the tofu (and reserved marinade if air-fried) and stir well for another couple of minutes. Serve with a side salad, if wished.

Nutrition per serving: 385kcal, Fat 18g, of which saturates 2.6g, Carbohydrates 19g, of which sugars 11g, Fibre 9.6g, Protein 31g

MAINS
Vegetarian and Vegan

Lentil Bolognese

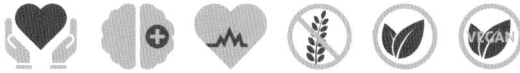

Rich and hearty, this lentil bolognese makes a delicious, healthy, comforting dish. Lentils are packed with B vitamins, magnesium, zinc and potassium as well as plenty of fibre and protein to support heart health and boost energy levels.

Preparation time: 15 minutes

Cooking time: 25 minutes

Serves 2

Ingredients

- 15g porcini mushrooms
- 2 tsp olive oil
- ½ onion, finely diced
- 1 garlic clove, crushed
- 1 celery stalk, diced
- 1 small carrot, diced
- 6 button mushrooms, diced
- ½ tsp smoked paprika
- Pinch of chilli powder
- Pinch of sea salt and black pepper
- 1 x 400g can brown lentils, drained and rinsed
- 1 vegetable stock cube
- 1 x 400g can chopped tomatoes
- 1 tbsp tomato puree
- 120g dried wholegrain or lentil pasta

To serve: Chopped parsley

Method

Soak the dried mushrooms in 50ml boiled water for 10 minutes and then drain, reserving the water. Finely chop.

Heat the oil in a large saucepan and sauté the onion, garlic, celery and carrot for 5 minutes. Add the mushrooms, paprika, chilli, salt, pepper, lentils, porcini mushroom and reserved liquid, tomatoes, tomato puree and stock cube. Stir well and simmer covered, for 20 minutes.

MAINS
Vegetarian and Vegan

Meanwhile cook the pasta according to packet instructions and drain. Garnish with chopped parsley and serve with the pasta. Accompany with a mixed salad.

Nutrition per serving: 487kcal, Fat 8.5g, of which saturates 1.4, Carbohydrates 68g, of which sugars 17g, Fibre 20g, Protein 22g

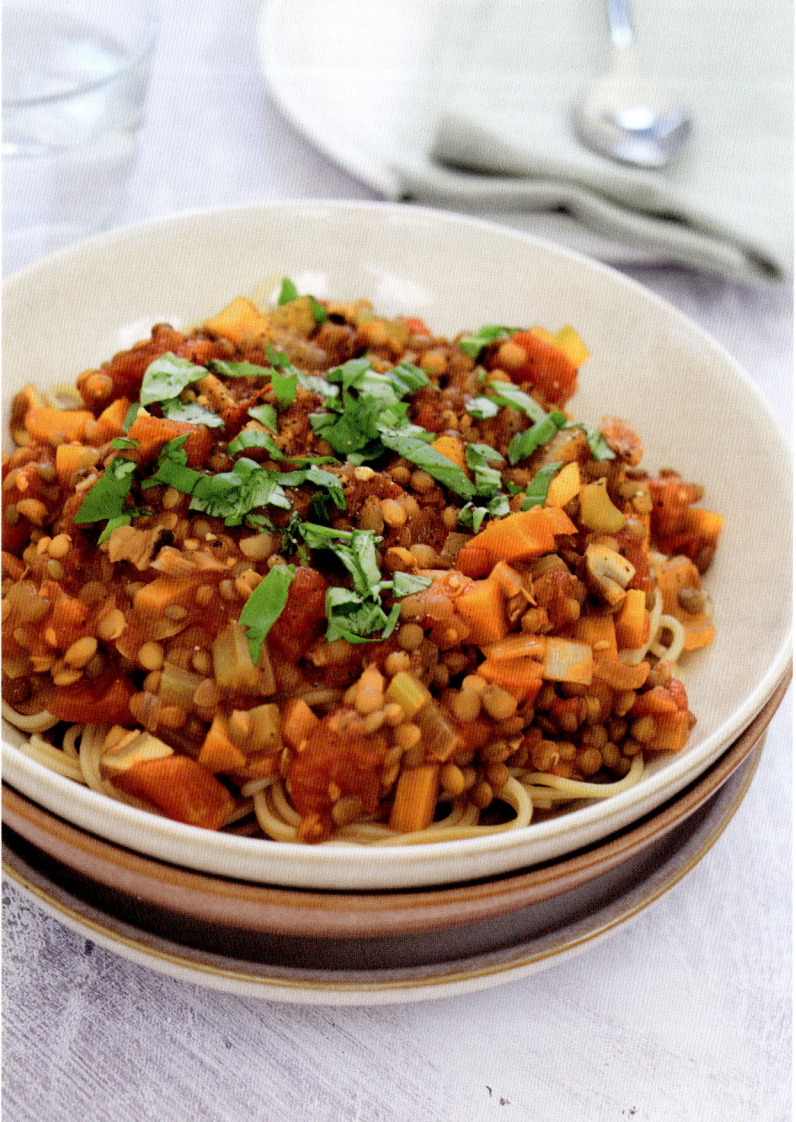

Baked Creamy Dahl with Tomatoes and Spinach

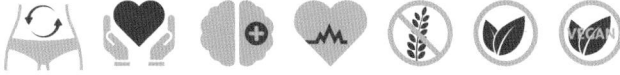

Baking dahl in the oven makes this a no-fuss dish and perfect for busy days. With the addition of anti-inflammatory turmeric and creamy coconut, this is a delicious creamy version. Lentils are a great source of fibre, which can help reduce hunger and balance blood sugar levels, making them ideal for managing a healthy weight. Accompany with a side salad if wished.

Preparation time: 15 minutes

Cooking time: 50 minutes

Serves 2

Ingredients

- 1 tbsp olive oil
- 1 onion, diced
- 1 garlic clove, crushed
- ¾ tsp ground turmeric
- 1 tsp ground cumin
- 1 tsp ground coriander
- 150g red lentils, rinsed
- 1 x 400ml tin light coconut milk
- 200ml boiling water
- 150g cherry tomatoes, halved
- 100g baby spinach leaves
- 2 limes, juice and zest
- Sea salt flakes, to taste

Method

Place the olive oil in a large casserole dish (with a lid) and sauté the onion and garlic for 5 minutes, to soften. Add the spices, lentils, coconut milk and water, and stir well. Bring to the boil then cover and place in the oven for 40 minutes.

Remove from the oven and place on the hob. Stir in the tomatoes, spinach and lime juice and zest, and cook gently for a further 5 minutes, to soften the tomatoes. Season to taste.

> **Nutrition per serving:** 524kcal, Fat 23g, of which saturates 14g, Carbohydrates 45g, of which sugars 8g, Fibre 17g, Protein 24g

MAINS
Vegetarian and Vegan

Vegan Bibimbap Bowl

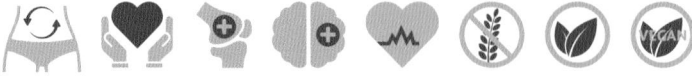

Bibimbap is a hot bowl of rice topped with various individually prepared, seasoned vegetables, with protein of choice. It is flavoured with a Gochujang (a Korean chilli paste) dressing to create a rich spicy dish. This colourful dish provides plenty of antioxidants and fibre, while the tofu is a good source of protein and phytoestrogens.

Preparation time: 15 minutes, plus marinating time

Cooking time: 20 minutes

Serves 2

Ingredients

- 350g firm tofu
- 1 tbsp tamari soy sauce
- 1 tsp mirin
- 1 tsp Gochujang (Korean chilli paste)
- 2 tsp olive oil, plus extra if frying tofu
- 150g shiitake mushrooms, sliced
- 2 baby pak choi, halved
- Handful of bean sprouts
- 1 small carrot, grated or shredded
- 60g cooked edamame beans
- 100g basmati rice cooked
- 1 tsp sesame seeds
- Toasted nori strips to garnish

Dressing

- 2 tsp Gochujang (Korean chilli paste)
- 2 tsp rice wine vinegar
- 1 tbsp tamari soy sauce
- 1 tsp brown sugar
- 1 small garlic clove, crushed

Method

Cut the tofu into cubes and place in a shallow bowl. Mix together the tamari soy sauce, mirin and Gochujang paste and pour over the tofu. Toss well to coat. If possible, leave for 30 minutes to marinate. Air-fry the tofu until golden (about 6–7 minutes) or pan-fry in a little oil for 5–6 minutes. Meanwhile, cook the rice according to the instructions.

Whisk all the dressing ingredients together.

Heat the olive oil in a frying pan. Add the shiitake mushrooms and sauté for 3–4 minutes, until softened. Remove from the pan. Add the pak choi with a splash of water and cook for 3–4 minutes, to soften. Remove from the pan. Add the bean sprouts and stir for a couple of minutes, to soften.

Divide the cooked rice between two bowls and top with the grated carrot, edamame beans and tofu. Drizzle over the dressing. Scatter over sesame seeds and strips of toasted nori, if wished.

Nutrition per serving: 447kcal, Fat 19g, of which saturates 2.6g, Carbohydrates 35g, of which sugars 16g, Fibre 9.6g, Protein 27g

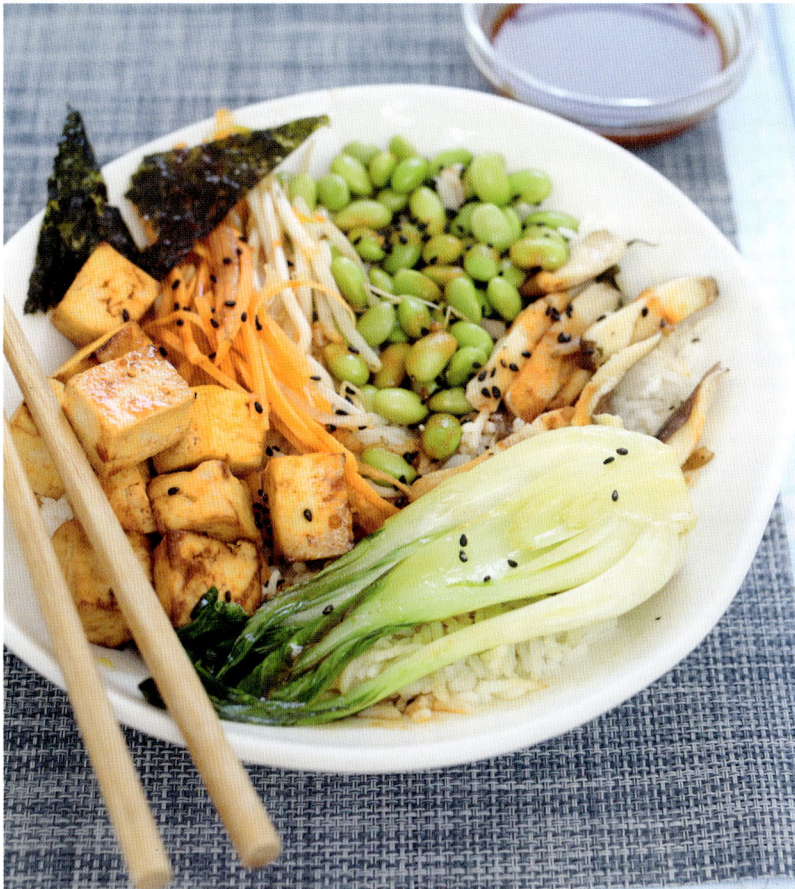

Tempeh San Choy Bow

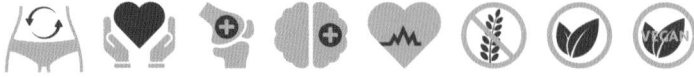

This is a vegan version of Chinese san choy bow. Crumbled tempeh makes a 'meaty' filling coated in a tangy dressing, while vegetables provide plenty of colour and texture. Tempeh is a fermented soy product and a good source of B vitamins, calcium, magnesium and iron. Rich in prebiotics and probiotics, it is an easily digestive protein that benefits digestive health.

Preparation time: 15 minutes

Cooking time: 9 minutes

Serves 2

Ingredients

- 2 tsp olive oil
- 300g tempeh, crumbled
- 100g button mushrooms, finely chopped
- ½ red onion, finely chopped
- 1 tsp freshly grated ginger
- 1 garlic clove, crushed
- ½ red chilli, deseeded and chopped
- 1 spring onion, finely sliced
- 4 canned water chestnuts, chopped
- 1 tbsp tamari soy sauce
- 1 tsp lime juice
- 1 tbsp vegan oyster sauce (or regular oyster sauce)
- 2 tbsp mirin
- Pinch of Chinese five-spice powder
- 1 tbsp sweet chilli sauce
- 1 tbsp coriander leaves
- 1 tbsp fresh mint leaves, chopped
- 4 iceberg lettuce cups or little gem leaves

Method

Heat the oil in a large frying pan over a medium heat. Add the tempeh and mushrooms and stir-fry for 3–4 minutes, until the mushrooms have reduced in size and are starting to turn golden.

Add the onion, ginger and garlic and stir well. Cook for another minute. Add the chilli, spring onion, water chestnuts, tamari, lime juice, oyster sauce, mirin, Chinese five-spice and sweet chilli sauce, and stir well to combine.

Stir through the fresh herbs. Spoon some of the mixture into iceberg lettuce leaves, wrap up and enjoy.

Nutrition per serving: 397kcal, Fat 14g, of which saturates 2.6g, Carbohydrates 26g, of which sugars 15g, Fibre 8.7g, Protein 35g

MAINS

Vegetarian and Vegan

Buckwheat, Fruit and Seed Bread

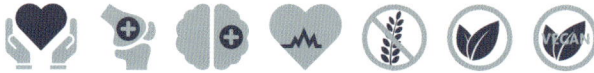

Packed with phytoestrogens, fibre and healthy fats, this is an ideal bread for a snack or breakfast/lunch option. Buckwheat is rich in magnesium, making it ideal for supporting your stress response, as well as being beneficial for bone and muscle health. This is best served on the day it is made, but it can also be sliced and then frozen.

Preparation time: 10 minutes, plus overnight soaking

Cooking time: 50 minutes

Makes 1 loaf/10 slices

Ingredients

- 60g buckwheat
- 30g ground flaxseed
- 50g chia seeds
- 100g buckwheat flour
- 1 tsp bicarbonate of soda
- 1 tsp baking powder
- 1 tsp ground cinnamon
- 300ml water
- 1 tbsp olive oil
- 1 tbsp powdered psyllium husks
- ½ tsp sea salt
- 1 tbsp apple cider vinegar
- 1 tbsp caster sugar, honey or maple syrup
- 30g pistachio nuts, shelled
- 50g dried fruit (raisins, cherries, etc.)

Method

Place the buckwheat in a bowl and cover with cold water. Leave to soak overnight, then drain and rinse well.

Preheat the oven to 160°C/Gas Mark 3. Grease a 1lb loaf tin and line with baking parchment.

Place the buckwheat in a food processor with the flaxseed, chia seeds and buckwheat flour, and process to combine. Add the remaining ingredients (except the nuts and dried fruit) and blend until smooth. Pulse in the pistachio nuts and dried fruit. Pour the mixture into the prepared loaf tin and smooth the top. Bake in the oven for 50 minutes, until a skewer or sharp knife inserted into the loaf comes out clean.

Turn out on to a rack and allow to cool before slicing.

> **Nutrition per serving/slice:** 149kcal, Fat 5.9g, of which saturates 0.8g, Carbohydrates 17g, of which sugars 5.1g, Fibre 5.3g, Protein 3.9g

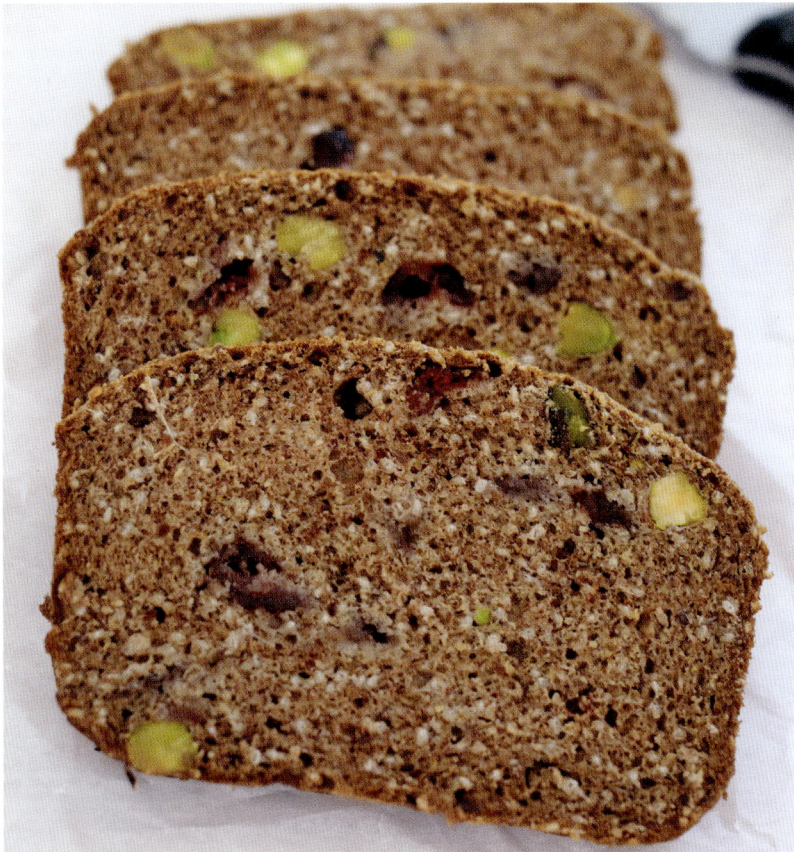

Cranberry Cottage Cheese Bread

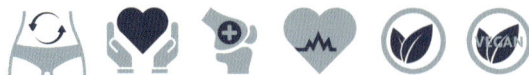

This is one of the simplest bread recipes ever, and thanks to the addition of cottage cheese, it has higher protein than traditional breads. It is delicious on its own or with butter or nut butter.

Preparation time: 10 minutes

Cooking time: 60 minutes

Makes 1 loaf/8 slices

Ingredients

- 200g oats (or gluten-free oats)
- 300g cottage cheese
- 40g dried cranberries, roughly chopped
- 1 tbsp mixed seeds
- 1 tsp cinnamon
- ½ tbsp baking powder (check GF if needed)
- 2 medium eggs, lightly beaten

Method

Preheat the oven to 180°C/Gas Mark 4. Line a baking tray with baking parchment.

Place all the ingredients in a mixing bowl and mix thoroughly together to form a dough. Turn out the dough and form into an oval shape, with floured hands. Place on a baking tray and bake for 50–60 minutes, until golden and cooked through. Allow to cool, then slice and serve. You can freeze this bread for up to 3 months.

Nutrition per serving/slice: 177kcal, Fat 6.5g, of which saturates 2g, Carbohydrates 20g, of which sugars 3.1g, Fibre 2.3g, Protein 9.1g

Tomato Flaxseed Crackers

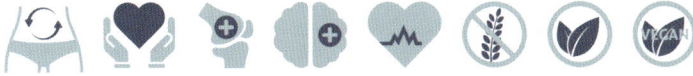

Flaxseeds are rich in phytoestrogens known as lignans, which may help alleviate symptoms such as hot flushes. Being a good source of soluble fibre they can be helpful for lowering cholesterol and supporting digestive health. These light, crunchy crackers are delicious served with dips or as an accompaniment to soups and salads.

Preparation time: 15 minutes

Cooking time: 25 minutes

Makes around 20–24 crackers

Ingredients

- 300g whole flaxseed
- 2 tomatoes, chopped
- 6 sundried tomatoes in oil, drained and chopped
- 2 tbsp lemon juice
- 2 tbsp nutritional yeast flakes
- ½ tsp sea salt
- 185ml water
- oil for greasing

Method

Line a baking tray with non-stick parchment paper and lightly oil. Lightly oil another piece of baking parchment the same size. Preheat the oven to 200°C/Gas Mark 6.

Grind the flaxseed in a food processor until fine. Add the remaining ingredients and blend to form a stiff paste. Use enough water to create a thick spreadable dough. Spread the dough on to one of the sheets of baking parchment with your fingers. Place the other baking parchment sheet on top, oiled-side down, and roll out the dough. Remove the top parchment. Place the dough on the baking sheet. Score lines into the dough to make individual crackers.

Bake for 18–20 minutes, until the crackers are lightly browned. Flip them over and gently peel off the parchment. Return to the oven for a further 5 minutes, to crisp up the crackers. Cool completely before breaking into individual crackers along the score lines.

Nutrition per cracker: 68kcal, Fat 5.5g, of which saturates 0.5g, Carbohydrates 0.6g, of which sugars 0.6g, Fibre 3.9g, Protein 2g

Salt and Vinegar Roasted Chickpeas

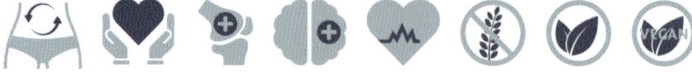

Oven-roasted chickpeas are super-simple to make, and are a delicious, crispy, high-protein snack. They can also be air-fried. Being naturally high in fibre and protein, they are a great way to help with reducing hunger and supporting healthy blood sugar. Chickpeas are incredibly nutritious, rich in B vitamins, iron, zinc, magnesium, copper and manganese, useful for boosting energy.

Preparation time: 10 minutes

Cooking time: 30 minutes

Serves 6 as a snack

Ingredients

- 1 x 400g can chickpeas, drained and rinsed
- 200ml white wine vinegar
- 1 tbsp olive oil
- 1 tsp sea salt

Method

Place the chickpeas in a small, shallow pan with the vinegar. Bring to a simmer, then turn off the heat and allow the chickpeas to soak for 30 minutes. Drain and discard the vinegar.

Preheat the oven to 200°C/Gas Mark 6.

Place the drained chickpeas on a clean kitchen towel and pat dry. It is important for the chickpeas to be as dry as possible before they hit the oven. Place the chickpeas on a baking tray and drizzle over the olive oil. Add the salt and toss until evenly distributed.

Roast for around 30 minutes, stirring occasionally. They should be golden and crisp. Allow to cool before eating. Alternatively, you can air-fry the chickpeas for 10–15 minutes until crisp. Shake occasionally during cooking.

> **Nutrition per serving:** 67kcal, Fat 3.2g, of which saturates 0.4g, Carbohydrates 6g, of which sugars 0g, Fibre 1.5g, Protein 2.8g

Chocolate-Coated Chickpeas

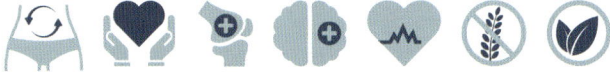

This is another great way of using chickpeas as a snack. This time they are baked and then coated in chocolate, to make a deliciously sweet treat.

Preparation time: 10 minutes

Cooking time: 42 minutes

Freezing time: 15 minutes

Serves 6 as a snack

Ingredients

- 1 x 400g can chickpeas, drained
- 100g dark chocolate (for vegan check labels)
- 1 tsp coconut oil

Method

Preheat the oven to 180°C/Gas Mark 4.

Rinse the chickpeas under cold water, then place on a baking tray lined with greaseproof paper. Rub the chickpeas with kitchen towel to lightly dry them. Place in the oven and roast for 40 minutes, turning them occasionally. Allow to cool for 10 minutes.

Break up the chocolate into a pan and add the coconut oil. Melt, stirring throughout, over a gentle heat. Add the chickpeas and stir well. If you wish, add a pinch of sea salt.

Place a piece of non-stick parchment on a small freezer-proof tray. Spread out the chickpea mixture. Alternatively, scoop out the mixture a tablespoon at a time to make clusters, leaving a little space between each cluster. Place in the freezer to harden – about 15 minutes. Remove from the freezer and place in the fridge, ready for snacking.

Nutrition per serving: 154kcal, Fat 8.8g, of which saturates 5g, Carbohydrates 12g, of which sugars 4.8g, Fibre 4.6g, Protein 4.7g

SWEET AND SAVOURY
SNACKS AND SIDES

DESSERTS AND SWEET TREATS

Berry Yogurt Granola Pots

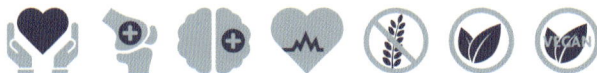

Simple to put together, these granola pots make an ideal sweet treat or breakfast option. Naturally sweet, they are a great source of antioxidants and vitamin C as well as probiotics to support digestive health and immune function.

Preparation time: 10 minutes

Cooking time: 4 minutes

Serves 2

Ingredients

- 200g mixed frozen berries
- 1 tsp cornflour mixed into 1 tbsp water
- Zest and juice of ½ orange
- 120g Greek yogurt (or dairy-free yogurt)
- 100g granola (see Chai Spiced Granola, page 142)

Method

Place the frozen berries in a small pan with the cornflour mixture. Simmer gently for 3–4 minutes, stirring with a wooden spoon to break up the fruit a little. Stir the orange zest and juice into the yogurt. To assemble, spoon the fruit compote into the bottom of two glasses. Top with yogurt and then the granola.

Nutrition per serving: 273kcal, Fat 16g, of which saturates 3g, Carbohydrates 23g, of which sugars 14g, Fibre 5.7g, Protein 6.3g

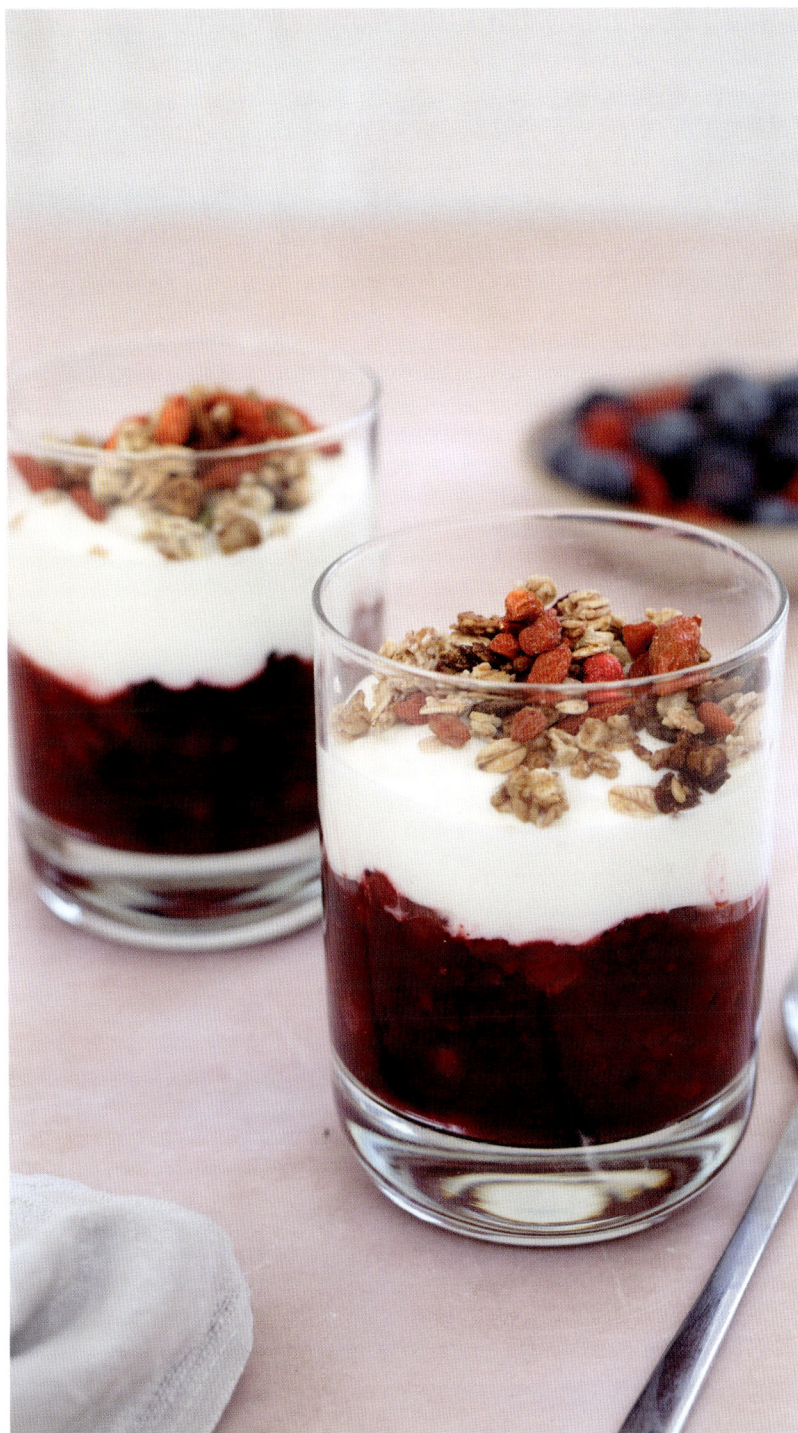

Baked Peaches with Elderflower Yogurt

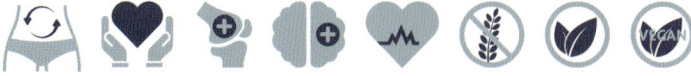

Baking fruit naturally sweetens and intensifies their flavour. Peaches are a good source of vitamins C and A to support skin health and immune function, plus fibre to help digestive health and balance blood sugar levels.

Preparation time: 10 minutes

Cooking time: 18 minutes

Serves 2

Ingredients

- 2 peaches or nectarines
- Zest and juice of ½ orange
- 1 tbsp honey
- 2 star anise

Yogurt

- 150g natural yogurt (or dairy-free yogurt)
- 1 tbsp elderflower cordial

Method

Mix the yogurt with the elderflower in a small bowl.

Preheat the oven to 180°C/Gas Mark 4.

Halve and stone the peaches, then cut each of the halves into two. Place the fruit in a roasting tin so they fit snugly. Squeeze the orange juice over and then drizzle with the honey and scatter over the zest. Add the star anise to the tin. Cover lightly with foil and roast for 15 minutes – the fruit should be soft, but still hold its shape.

Preheat the grill to high. Remove the foil and grill for 2–3 minutes until golden. Serve with the yogurt.

> **Nutrition per serving:** 120kcal, Fat 0.9g, of which saturates 0.5g, Carbohydrates 22g, of which sugars 21g, Fibre 2.3g, Protein 4.8g

Matcha Green Tea Mint Ice Cream

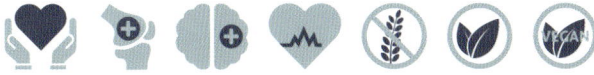

Adding silken tofu to this ice cream recipe creates a wonderful smooth, creamy texture, as well as boosting its protein content. Matcha is rich in catechins, a class of plant compounds in tea that act as natural antioxidants, helping to lower inflammation and protect the body from cell damage. Matcha has been shown to improve attention, memory and reaction time. It also contains caffeine and L-theanine, which can improve several aspects of brain function.

Preparation time: 15 minutes

Freezing time: 3–4 hours

Serves 4

Ingredients

- 350g silken tofu, drained
- 1 tbsp matcha green tea powder
- 30g vanilla protein powder
- 60g caster sugar (or sweetener of choice)
- Handful of fresh mint leaves
- 250ml light or full-fat coconut milk
- Dash of peppermint extract, to taste
- 30g coconut oil, softened

Method

Simply place all the ingredients in a high-speed blender and process until smooth and creamy. Pour the mixture into an ice cream machine and churn according to the instructions, and then freeze until required. Alternatively, pour the mixture into a shallow freezer-proof container and place in the freezer for 3–4 hours, until firm. Remove from the freezer about 10 minutes before serving to allow the ice cream to soften slightly.

Nutrition per serving: 261kcal, Fat 15g, of which saturates 11g, Carbohydrates 19g, of which sugars 17g, Fibre 1.9g, Protein 12g

DESSERTS AND SWEET TREATS

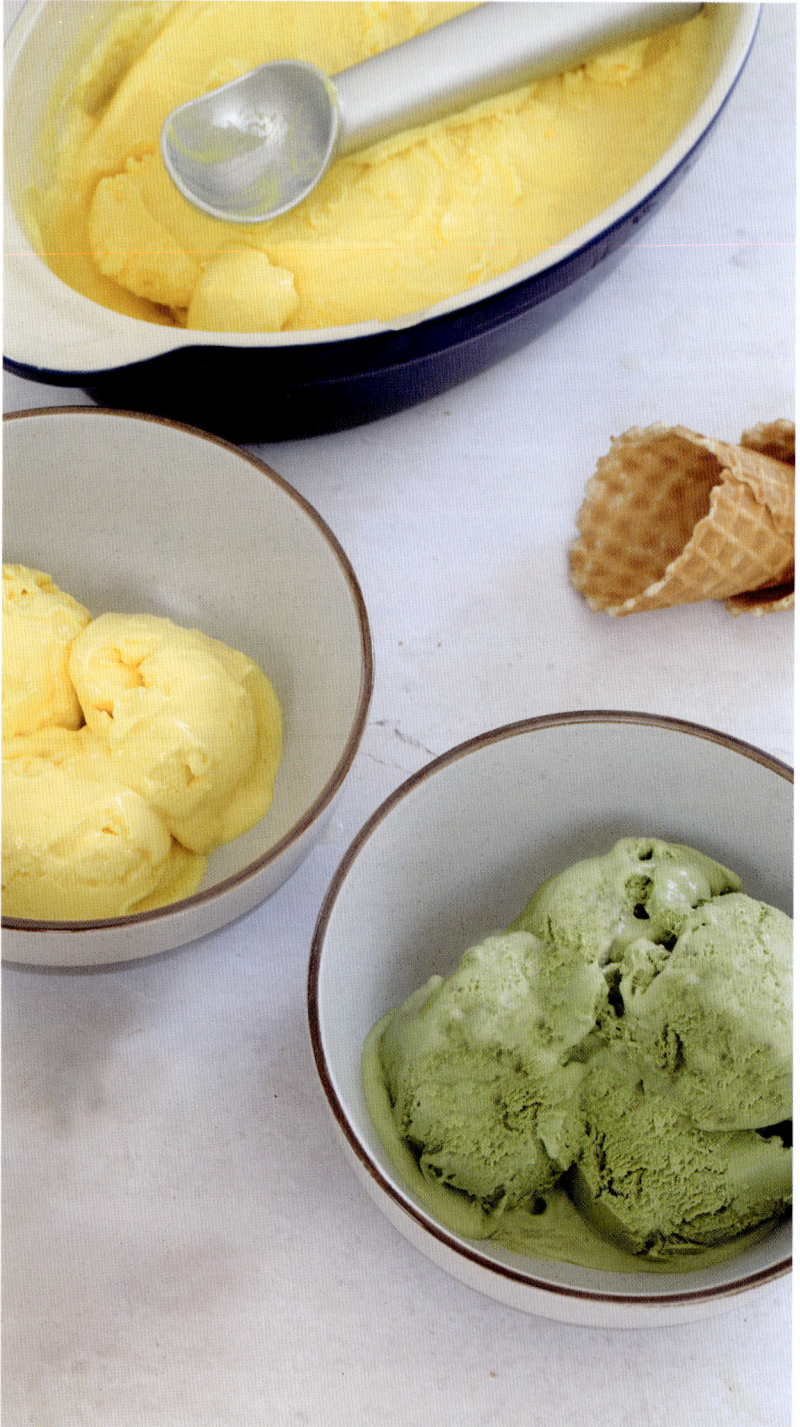

Mango Protein Ice Cream

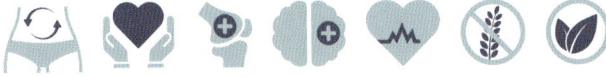

Light and fruity, this mango ice cream is rich in B vitamins, calcium and protein, yet low in added sugars. It is a delicious, healthy treat.

Preparation time: 10 minutes

Freezing time: 3–4 hours

Serves 4

Ingredients

- 300g cottage cheese
- 250g frozen mango
- 1 tbsp honey or maple syrup (or sweetener of choice)
- 1 tbsp protein powder (optional)

Method

In a high-speed blender or food processor, combine all the ingredients and blend until smooth. You can serve this immediately, although it will be a little soft, or you can transfer the mixture to a shallow container and freeze until firm (about 3–4 hours). Then let the ice cream sit at room temperature for 10 minutes before serving.

Nutrition per serving: 121kcal, **Fat** 4.9g, of which saturates 2.5g, Carbohydrates 12g, of which sugars 12g, Fibre 0.7g, Protein 7.3g

Chocolate Maca Tart

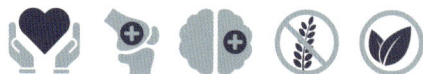

This is a delicious, high-protein and low-sugar dessert. Easy to prepare, it can be frozen ahead of time, making it perfect for a special treat. Maca is an adaptogenic herb, which may boost energy and mood and ease hot flashes in some postmenopausal women.

Preparation time: 15 minutes

Chilling time: 4 hours

Serves 12

Ingredients
Base

- 140g regular oats (or gluten-free oats)
- 50g hazelnuts
- 50g soft dried fruit (if hard, soak in hot water first, then drain)
- 50g butter (or dairy-free spread), melted

Filling

- 300g dark chocolate (or vegan chocolate), melted
- 350g silken tofu
- 200g Greek yogurt (or soy yogurt)
- 1 scoop chocolate protein powder or 1 tbsp cocoa powder
- 2–3 tsp maca powder, to taste
- Pinch of salt
- 1 tbsp honey or maple syrup

To decorate: Fresh or freeze-dried berries, chocolate shavings or cacao nibs

Method

Place the ingredients for the base in a food processor and blitz until the mixture comes together. Tip into a lined 20cm/8 inch cake tin with a removable base and press down firmly.

Place all the ingredients for the filling into a blender and process until smooth. Pour the mixture over the base and smooth the top. Place in the fridge and chill for 4 hours, or place in the freezer until firm.

Remove from the cake tin, then decorate with berries and a little grated chocolate or cacao nibs. Cut into slices to serve.

Nutrition per serving: 285kcal, Fat 18g, of which saturates 7.5g, Carbohydrates 21g, of which sugars 11g, Fibre 4.3g, Protein 8.4g

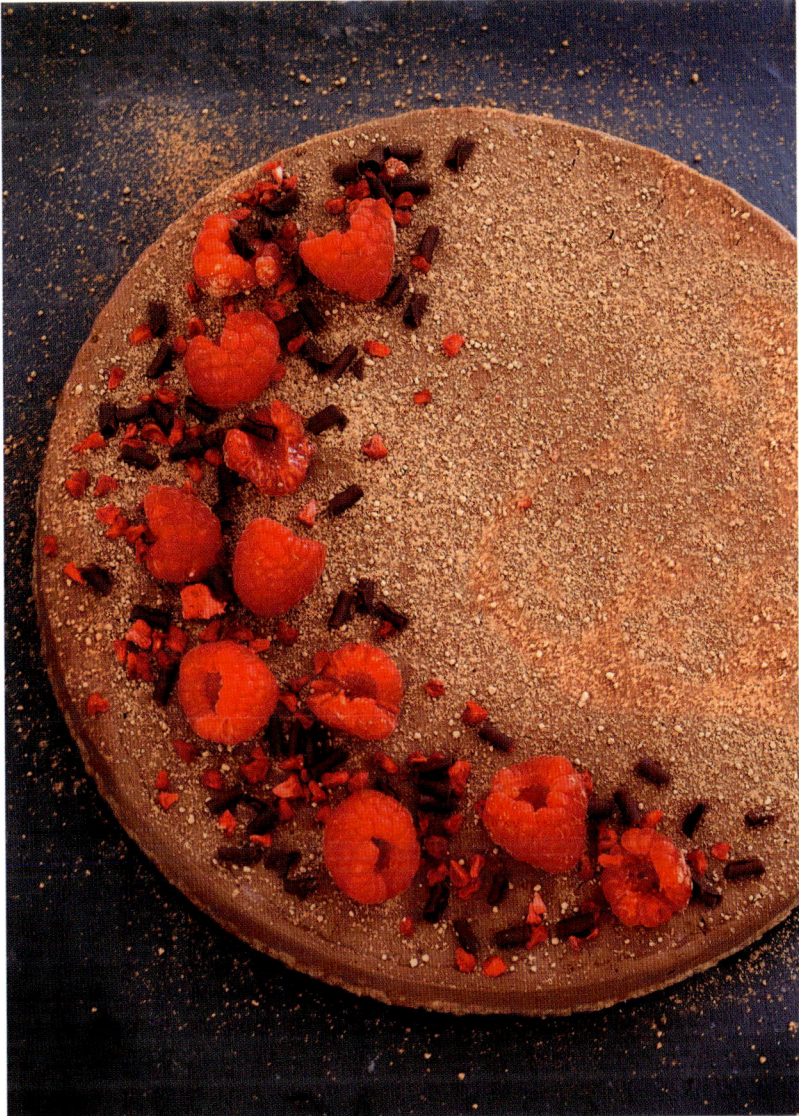

Baked Lemon Cheesecake with Berry Compote

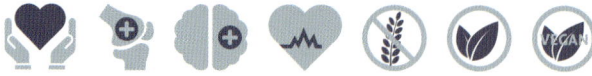

Rich and creamy, this cheesecake is lower in saturated fat than traditional versions, thanks to the use of silken tofu instead of a cream-based filling. Serve with a berry compote for additional protective antioxidants. A good source of protein, fibre, calcium plus phytoestrogens makes this a wonderful, healthy dessert.

Preparation time: 15 minutes

Cooking time: 50 minutes

Serves 12

Ingredients
Base

- 200g plain flour (or gluten-free flour; if using gluten-free flour add ¼ tsp xanthum)
- ½ tsp salt
- ½ tsp baking powder
- 30g caster sugar
- 140g butter (or vegan butter)
- 1–2 tbsp water, to bind

Filling

- 700g silken tofu, drained
- 125ml Greek yogurt (or soy yogurt)
- 50g butter (or vegan butter), melted
- Juice and zest of 1 lemon
- 50g cornflour
- 100g caster sugar (or sweetener of choice)

Berry compote

- 300g frozen berries (blueberries or a mixture)
- 2 tbsp cornflour, dissolved in 2 tbsp water
- sugar (optional)

Method

Preheat the oven to 180°C/Gas Mark 4. Grease and line a 20cm/8 inch spring-form cake tin.

Place the ingredients for the base in a food processor and blend well. Add 1–2 tbsp water and continue to process until the mixture comes together to form a soft dough – it should be quite damp. Transfer the dough to the lined cake tin and press over the base and a little up the sides – you may find it easier to do this with damp hands. Place in the fridge while you make the filling.

Place all the ingredients for the filling in a food processor and blend until really smooth and creamy. Pour the filling over the base and bake in the oven for 45–50 minutes, until lightly golden and the middle is set. Remove from the oven and allow to cool completely. Place in the fridge.

For the compote, place the berries in a small pan with the cornflour and a little sugar if wished, and stir well for a couple of minutes to break down the fruit to form a thick compote. Serve the cheesecake with the berry compote spooned over.

Nutrition per serving: 286kcal, Fat 15g, of which saturates 7.4g, Carbohydrates 34g, of which sugars 14g, Fibre 1.5g, Protein 4.4g

DESSERTS AND SWEET TREATS

Apple Oat Slices

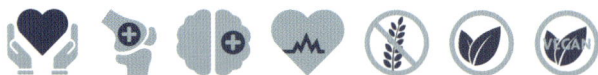

Low in added sugar, these oat slices are rich in fibre, which can increase the feeling of fullness, making them useful when trying to lose weight. Apples also contain polyphenols that may support heart health and a healthy gut microbiome. You could use prepared apple puree instead, if wished. Alternatively, any fruit could work well as the filling.

Preparation time: 15 minutes

Cooking time: 30 minutes

Makes 16 slices

Ingredients
Filling

- 8 eating apples, cored and diced
- 2 tbsp water
- Juice and zest of ½ lemon
- Pinch of ground cinnamon
- 30g butter

Base and topping

- 120g coconut oil or butter, melted
- 50g peanut butter or almond nut butter
- 3 tbsp honey or maple syrup
- 250g porridge oats (or gluten-free oats)
- 1 tsp baking powder
- Pinch of salt
- 1 tsp cinnamon
- 30g desiccated coconut

Method

Preheat the oven to 180°C/Gas Mark 4. Grease and line a 20cm/8 inch square baking tin.

First, make the filling. Add the apples to a pan with the water. Simmer for 2–3 minutes to soften the fruit, then add the rest of the ingredients and cook on a low heat for 2–3 minutes, until the fruit is very soft and forms a thick puree. Set aside.

For the base, gently melt the coconut oil, peanut butter and honey in a pan. In a food processor add the oats, baking powder, salt, cinnamon, and desiccated coconut and mix briefly. Add the coconut oil mixture and mix to combine. You want to keep some texture, so do not overprocess.

Transfer two-thirds of the oat mixture into the baking tin and press down firmly. Spread the apple puree on top, then crumble the remaining oat mixture over the top and press it down gently into the puree.

Bake for 25–30 minutes until golden. Cool completely in the tin, then place in the fridge to chill before cutting into bars.

Nutrition per slice: 214kcal, Fat 13g, of which saturates 9.1g, Carbohydrates 19g, of which sugars 8.2g, Fibre 2.4g, Protein 3.3g

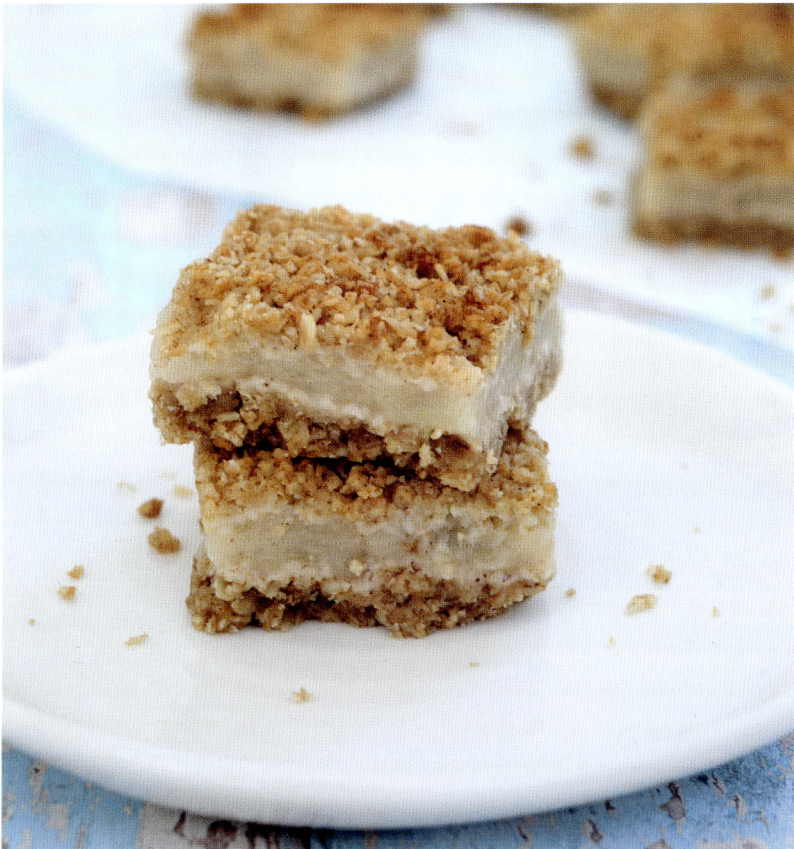

Protein Lemon and Poppy Seed Mug Cake

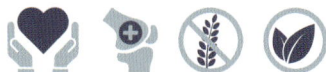

Mug cakes are perfect for when you fancy something quick and sweet. These lemon and poppy seed cakes contain added protein powder for a protein boost. Poppy seeds are particularly rich in manganese, a trace element important for bone health.

Preparation time: 5 minutes

Cooking time: 2 minutes

Serves 1

Ingredients

- 2 tbsp plain flour (or gluten-free flour)
- 1 tbsp vanilla protein powder
- ½ tsp baking powder (check GF if needed)
- Pinch of salt
- 1 egg
- 1 tsp lemon zest
- 1 tbsp lemon juice
- 1 tsp caster sugar (or sweetener of choice)
- ½ tsp poppy seeds
- 2 tbsp milk (or milk alternative)
- oil for greasing

To serve: Yogurt

Method

Lightly grease a mug with a little oil. Add all the ingredients to the mug and mix well together, to form a thick batter. Microwave on high for 1–2 minutes. Alternatively, to oven bake, place in a preheated oven (180°C/Gas Mark 4) and bake for 20 minutes, or air-fry for around 8 minutes.

> **Nutrition per serving:** 267kcal, Fat 7.9g, of which saturates 2.1g, Carbohydrates 30g, of which sugars, 5.8g, Fibre 2.8g, Protein 17g

Lemon Blueberry Oat Muffins

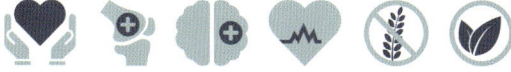

These are delicious, reduced-sugar muffins, full of slow-releasing carbohydrates and nutritious seeds. This is a perfect healthy option for breakfast, but equally delicious as a grab-and-go snack.

Preparation time: 10 minutes

Cooking time: 20 minutes

Makes 8 muffins

Ingredients

- 150g self-raising flour (or gluten-free self-raising flour)
- 2 tsp baking powder
- 1 tbsp ground flaxseed
- Pinch of sea salt
- 1 tsp cinnamon
- 100g porridge oats or muesli (or gluten-free oats)
- 60g caster sugar
- 3 eggs
- 4 tbsp olive oil
- Zest of 1 lemon and 1 tbsp lemon juice
- 125ml milk (or milk alternative)
- 100g fresh blueberries

Method

Preheat the oven to 180°C/Gas Mark 4. Line a muffin tray with cases.

Place the flour, baking powder, flaxseed, sea salt, cinnamon, oats or muesli and sugar in a large mixing bowl, with the lemon zest.

Beat the eggs, olive oil, lemon juice and milk in a jug. Pour into the flour mixture and beat well to form a thick batter. Stir in the blueberries, gently.

Spoon the mixture into the muffin cases. Bake for 20 minutes, until golden brown and firm on top. Leave to cool in the tins for 5–10 minutes before turning out and cooling on a rack.

Nutrition per muffin: 247kcal, Fat 9.9g, of which saturates 1.8g, Carbohydrates 32g, of which sugars 9.5g, Fibre 2.2g, Protein 6.6g

DESSERTS AND SWEET TREATS

Tahini Miso Swirl Brownies

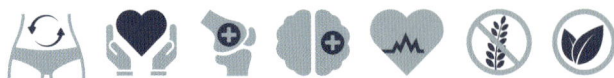

Tahini is a nutritious paste made from ground sesame seeds. It is particularly rich in copper, which is useful for iron absorption, and selenium that helps lower inflammation and support immune health. Sesame seeds are a source of phytoestrogens, which may help alleviate hot flushes.

Preparation time: 10 minutes

Cooking time: 25 minutes

Makes 16 brownies

Ingredients
Brownie

- 100g butter (or dairy-free spread)
- 200g dark chocolate
- 75g caster sugar (or sweetener of choice)
- 3 eggs
- 60ml milk (or soy milk)
- 1 tsp vanilla extract
- 100g self-raising flour (or gluten-free self-raising flour)
- ½ tsp baking powder
- ½ tsp bicarbonate of soda

Swirl

- 3 tbsp tahini
- 2 tsp white miso paste
- 2 tsp maple syrup
- 2 tbsp Greek yogurt (or soy yogurt)
- White sesame seeds for sprinkling (optional)

Method
Preheat the oven to 180°C/Gas Mark 4.

Place the butter, chocolate and sugar in a pan and warm gently to melt the chocolate. Cool slightly, then place the chocolate mixture in a food processor with the eggs, milk, vanilla, flour, baking powder and bicarbonate of soda, and process to combine.

Spoon the mixture into a square 20cm/8 inch baking tin.

Mix together the tahini, miso, maple syrup and yogurt. Spoon dollops of the tahini mixture on to the brownie mixture and then use a knife or a chopstick to create a swirl effect.

Bake the brownies for 25 minutes, until golden and cooked through. Allow to cool in the tin and then cut into bars. Store in an airtight container for a week or in the fridge. They can be also be frozen for up to 3 months.

Nutrition per brownie: 196kcal, Fat 13g, of which saturates 7.1g, Carbohydrates 14g, of which sugars 8.4g, Fibre 2g, Protein 4g

Bone-Boosting Slice

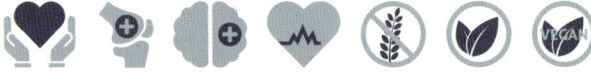

This fruit and nut slice makes a delicious, nutritious treat. It can be sliced and frozen in portions, making it an ideal grab-and-go option. Prunes are a fabulous bone-supporting food. Researchers have found that they can help prevent or delay bone loss in postmenopausal women, possibly due to their ability to reduce inflammation and oxidative stress, both of which contribute to bone loss.

Preparation time: 20 minutes, plus soaking time

Cooking time: 30 minutes

Makes 12–14 slices

Ingredients

- 250g dried, pitted soft prunes
- 2 tbsp tahini
- Juice of 1 orange
- 60g chopped almonds
- 60g chopped pistachio nuts
- 30g sunflower seeds
- 30g pumpkin seeds
- 40g puffed rice
- 30g ground flaxseed
- 1 tbsp maca powder
- Pinch of sea salt
- 30g vanilla or chocolate protein powder (optional)

Topping

- 300g dark chocolate chips
- 2 tsp coconut oil

Method

Line a 2lb loaf tin with parchment paper – allow the sides to hang over as this makes it easier to turn out. Preheat the oven to 150°C/Gas Mark 2.

Pour boiling water over the prunes and leave to soak for 20 minutes, then drain. Place the prunes in a food processor with the tahini and orange juice. Process to form a thick paste.

Place all the other ingredients in a large bowl and stir well. Add the prune mixture and, using your hands, massage it into the dry ingredients so they are completely coated.

Spread the mixture into the loaf tin. Press it down really well, so it is firm. Bake for about 30 minutes, until lightly golden. Remove from the oven and press the mixture down again, then allow to cool completely.

Melt the chocolate and coconut oil in a pan. Once the prune mixture is completely cool, pour over the chocolate and smooth the surface. Place in the fridge to set completely. Turn out and then slice to serve.

Nutrition per slice: 276kcal, Fat 19g, of which saturates 7.2g, Carbohydrates 18g, of which sugars 13g, Fibre 5.4g, Protein 6.2g

Protein Energy Bites

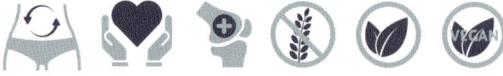

This is a great sweet snack, packed with protein and healthy fats to keep you energized through the day. Make up a batch of these and freeze them ready for a pick-me-up when energy levels are flagging.

Preparation time: 10 minutes

Chilling time: 30 minutes

Serves 2

Ingredients

- 60g oats (or gluten-free oats)
- 40g tahini or nut butter
- 30g protein powder (any flavour)
- 2 tsp vanilla extract
- 2 tsp honey or maple syrup
- Pinch of cinnamon, to taste

Method

In a food processor, add all the ingredients and pulse together until well combined. If the mixture is too dry, add a splash of water to form a sticky dough-like consistency. With clean hands take the mixture and roll them into 8 bite-sized balls. Place the balls on a tray and chill in the fridge for 30 minutes to firm up. They can also be frozen for up to three months.

Nutrition per bite: 79 kcal, Fat 3.7g, of which saturates 0.6g, Carbohydrates 5.6g, of which sugars 0.8g, Fibre 1.1g, Protein 5.2g

Appendix: Example Seven-Day Meal Plans

Our Reset meal plans are designed to help you lose weight and support a healthier body composition. They are higher in protein and lower in carbohydrates to help you feel fuller for longer, support muscle mass and improve blood glucose management. Protein is spread evenly throughout the day, with a focus on a higher intake at breakfast compared to typical meals. Research suggests this may be particularly beneficial for maintaining muscle mass. The plans are structured to support weight loss, but you can adjust portion sizes based on your activity level and individual goals.

The meal plans are deliberately simple and some make use of leftovers. The recipes are also ideal for batch cooking, meaning you can prepare the meals in advance and chill or freeze them. If you wish to bulk up any of the meals, you can add some non-starchy vegetables including cruciferous vegetables (e.g., broccoli, pak choi, cabbage, cauliflower) and leafy green salads. This will provide additional fibre to help stop you from feeling too hungry. For drinks, choose water, herbal teas, coffee, black or green tea. Add milk or milk alternatives if preferred but avoid all high-calorie sugary drinks.

To support improvements in body composition and insulin sensitivity, consider:

- *Protein powder*: You will notice that some of the recipes include protein powder. This is a convenient way to increase your daily protein intake. Alternatively, you can simply take it as a shake post workout or as a snack.
- Consider supplementation to enhance insulin sensitivity (see Chapter 3).

- *Exercise:* It is recommended to include at least one hour of steady-state exercise (e.g., walking, running, cycling, exercise class, dancing) and strength training at least 2–3 times a week (or more).

Note: Where the meal plans say mixed salad or vegetables, there is no oil dressing.

EXAMPLE 7-DAY RESET MEAL PLAN

Day	Breakfast	Lunch	Dinner	Snack
Sunday	Super Greens Smoothie	Mushroom and Herb Omelette with Salsa Verde and mixed salad	Smoky Chipotle Chicken with Chunky Guacamole Mixed salad	100g low-fat Greek yogurt (or soy yogurt) with 15g protein powder
Monday	Protein Overnight Oats	Leftover Smoky Chipotle Chicken with mixed salad	Traybake Salmon with Pak Choi and Tomatoes	Blueberry Brain Boost
Tuesday	Super Greens Smoothie	Chicken Panzanella Salad Piece of fruit	Baked Creamy Dahl with Tomatoes and Spinach Mixed salad	Chocolate Protein Pot
Wednesday	Protein Yogurt with Berries	Chicken Panzanella Salad Piece of fruit	One-Pan Beef and Lentil Chilli Mixed salad or steamed greens	Creamy Chocolate Shake
Thursday	Creamy Protein Smoothie Bowl	Leftover One-Pan Beef and Lentil Chilli	Fish Tacos with Pickled Red Onions Steamed greens	Tropical Immune Blast
Friday	Tofu and Spinach Scramble	Smoked Salmon with Avocado and Smashed Broad Beans 100g blueberries or a piece of fruit	Thai Green Chicken Curry Mixed salad	Protein yogurt and fruit

| Saturday | 2-egg omelette with spinach and mushrooms | Leftover Thai Green Chicken Curry

Mixed salad

Piece of fruit | Tofu Vegetable Medley

Mixed salad | Creamy Chocolate Shake |

EXAMPLE 7-DAY VEGAN RESET MEAL PLAN

Day	Breakfast	Lunch	Dinner	Snack
Sunday	Protein Overnight Oats	Creamy Kale Salad with Chopped Apple with 150g air-fried/cooked tofu	Baked Creamy Dahl with Tomatoes and Spinach Mixed salad	100g low-fat soy yogurt with 30g scoop of protein powder
Monday	Creamy Chocolate Shake	Leftover Baked Creamy Dahl with Tomatoes and Spinach Piece of fruit	Leftover Creamy Kale Salad with Chopped Apple Tofu and Spinach Scramble	100g soy yogurt with handful of blueberries
Tuesday	Super Greens Smoothie	Tofu Burrito Mixed salad Piece of fruit	Roasted Vegetables and Puy Lentils with Harissa Dressing Mixed salad	Chocolate Protein Pot
Wednesday	Chocolate Protein Pot	Roasted Vegetables and Puy Lentils with Harissa Dressing Mixed salad	Tempeh San Choy Bow with leafy greens 100g soy yogurt with piece of fruit	Tropical Immune Blast
Thursday	Protein Overnight Oats	Leftover Tempeh San Choy Bow with leafy salad	Thai Green Curry with Tofu	Blueberry Brain Boost

cont.

Day	Breakfast	Lunch	Dinner	Snack
Friday	Super Greens Smoothie	Thai Green Curry with Tofu Protein yogurt (soy) with berries	Baked Creamy Dahl with Tomatoes and Spinach Mixed salad	Tropical Immune Blast
Saturday	Tofu and Spinach Scramble	Baked Creamy Dahl with Tomatoes and Spinach Mixed salad	Tofu Vegetable Medley Mixed salad	100g low-fat soy yogurt with 30g scoop of protein powder

RENEW MEAL PLANS

The following meal plans are examples to nourish the body for long term health and wellbeing while still be high in protein.

BONE HEALTH

Day	Breakfast	Lunch	Dinner	Snack/ dessert
Sunday	Tofu and Spinach Scramble Greek yogurt with nuts and seeds	Creamy Kale Salad with Chopped Apple with 100g cooked chicken, fish or tempeh	Teriyaki Chicken Noodle Salad	Bone-Boosting Slice
Monday	Creamy Chocolate Shake	Leftover Teriyaki Chicken Noodle Salad Greek yogurt and fruit	Pan-Fried Tempeh with Sweet Soy Ginger Dressing	4 prunes with 100g Greek yogurt or soy yogurt
Tuesday	Scrambled Eggs with Spinach and Salsa Greek yogurt with granola	Roasted Broccoli and Fennel Soup Nut butter or cream cheese on oat cakes or Tomato Flaxseed Crackers	Fish Tacos with Pickled Red Onions Mixed salad	Peanut and Apricot Oat Slice

Wednesday	Cottage Cheese Fruit Bowl	Leftover Fish Tacos with Pickled Red Onions Mixed salad Greek yogurt and fruit	Roasted Broccoli and Fennel Soup Tofu and Spinach Scramble with wholegrain toast or pitta	Creamy Chocolate Shake
Thursday	Tropical Immune Blast	Smoked Salmon with Avocado and Smashed Broad Beans Protein Yogurt with Berries	Mushroom Shawarma with Tahini Yogurt Mixed green vegetables/ salad Yogurt with nuts and seeds	Bone-Boosting Slice
Friday	Super Greens Smoothie	Leftover Mushroom Shawarma with Tahini Yogurt	Baked Sea Bass with Gremolata and Fennel Salad New potatoes/ steamed broccoli Protein yogurt and berries	Protein Lemon and Poppy Seed Mug Cake Greek yogurt
Saturday	Buckwheat Pancakes with Blueberry Compote and Greek yogurt	Tom Yum Soup with kimchi Wholegrain roll or flaxseed crackers 4 prunes with 100g Greek yogurt or soy yogurt	One-Pan Beef and Lentil Chilli Bone boosting slice	Cinnamon Maca Shake

BRAIN HEALTH

Day	Breakfast	Lunch	Dinner	Snack/Dessert
Sunday	Blueberry Brain Boost	Tom Yum Soup with kimchi Protein Yogurt with Berries	Roasted Oriental Trout with new potatoes and steamed vegetables	Matcha Green Tea Ice Cream
Monday	Protein Overnight Oats	Leftover Roasted Oriental Trout Large mixed salad with beetroot	Moroccan Spiced Lamb Tagine Mixed vegetables	Greek yogurt with berries or pomegranate seeds
Tuesday	Cinnamon Maca Shake	Tom Yum Soup with kimchi Protein Yogurt with Berries	Leftover Moroccan Spiced Lamb Tagine Mixed vegetables	Chocolate Protein Pot
Wednesday	Scrambled Eggs with Spinach and Salsa	Mackerel, Roasted Beetroot and Potato Salad Greek yogurt with fruit	Pomegranate-Griddled Chicken with Aubergine Mixed salad	Matcha Green Tea Ice Cream
Thursday	Tropical Immune Blast	Mackerel, Roasted Beetroot and Potato Salad	Lentil Bolognese	Cinnamon Maka Shake
Friday	Tofu and Spinach Scramble	2-egg omelette with vegetables 100g Greek yogurt with handful of berries	Lentil Bolognese Mixed salad/mixed vegetables	Super Greens Smoothie
Saturday	Cottage Cheese with Berries and Seeds	Tofu and Spinach Scramble Wholegrain pitta with nut butter	Indonesian Fish Curry Mixed salad/mixed vegetables	Chocolate Maca Tart

HEART HEALTH

Day	Breakfast	Lunch	Dinner	Snack/dessert
Sunday	Tropical Immune Blast	Smashed Edamame Beans with Lemon and Capers Mixed salad	Smoked Salmon and Herb Fish Cakes Mixed salad	Protein Yogurt with Berries
Monday	Vanilla Berry Chia Pots	Leftover Smoked Salmon and Herb Fish Cakes Mixed salad	Minestrone Soup Salad Tomato Flax-seed Crackers or pitta Protein Yogurt with Berries	Super Greens Smoothie
Tuesday	Vanilla Berry Chia Pots	Minestrone Soup Salad Tomato Flaxseed Crackers or pitta Protein Yogurt with Berries	Smoky Chipotle Chicken with Chunky Guacamole Mixed salad/mixed vegetables	Chocolate-Coated Chickpeas
Wednesday	Scrambled Eggs with Spinach and Salsa	Tofu Burrito Salad Protein yogurt with fruit	Traybake Salmon with Pak Choi and Tomatoes Mixed salad/new potatoes	Berry Yogurt Granola Pots
Thursday	Tropical Immune Blast	Leftover Traybake Salmon with Pak Choi and Tomatoes Salad Peanut and Apricot Slice	Baked Creamy Dahl with Tomatoes and Spinach Mixed salad/mixed vegetables	Chocolate-Coated Chickpeas
Friday	Super Greens Smoothie	Leftover Baked Creamy Dahl with Tomatoes and Spinach	Oven-Baked Frittata with Roast Pepper Salad	Protein Yogurt with Berries
Saturday	Tofu and Spinach Scramble with wholegrain pitta or toast	Leftover Oven-Baked Frittata with Roast Pepper Salad	Vegan Bibimbap Bowl	Baked Lemon Cheesecake with Berry Compote

Endnotes

Part 1

1 Freeman, E.W. and Sherif, K. (2007) 'Prevalence of hot flushes and night sweats around the world: A systematic review.' *Climacteric: The Journal of the International Menopause Society* 10, 3, 197–214. doi: 10.1080/13697130601181486.

Chapter 1

1 Mendelsohn, M.E. and Karas, R.H. (1999) 'The protective effects of estrogen on the cardiovascular system.' *The New England Journal of Medicine* 340, 23,1801–1811. doi: 10.1056/NEJM199906103402306.

2 Mauvais-Jarvis, F., Clegg, D.J. and Hevener, A.L. (2013) 'The role of estrogens in control of energy balance and glucose homeostasis.' *Endocrine Reviews* 34, 3, 309-338. doi: 10.1210/er.2012-1055.

3 Davis, S.R., Lambrinoudaki, I., Lumsden, M., Mishra, G.D., *et al.* (2015) 'Menopause.' *Nature Reviews Disease Primers* 1, 15004. doi: 10.1038/nrdp.2015.4.

4 Dahlman-Wright, K., Cavailles, V., Fuqua, S.A., Jordan, V.C., *et al.* (2006) 'International Union of Pharmacology. LXIV. Estrogen receptors.' *Pharmacological Reviews* 58, 4, 773-781. doi: 10.1124/pr.58.4.8.

5 Bedell, S., Nachtigall, M. and Naftolin, F. (2014) 'The pros and cons of plant estrogens for menopause.' *The Journal of Steroid Biochemistry and Molecular Biology* 139, 225–236. doi: 10.1016/j.jsbmb.2012.12.004.

6 Morito, K., Aomori, T., Hirose, T., Kinjo, J., *et al.* (2002) 'Interaction of phytoestrogens with estrogen receptors alpha and beta (II).' *Biological & Pharmaceutical Bulletin* 25, 1, 48–52. doi: 10.1248/bpb.25.48.

7 Dimitrakakis, C., Zhou, J. and Bondy, C.A. (2002) 'Androgens and mammary growth and neoplasia.' *Fertility and Sterility* 77, Suppl. 4, 26–33. doi: 10.1016/S0015-0282(02)02979-5.

8 Panay, N. and Fenton, A. (2009) 'The role of testosterone in women.' *Climacteric* 12, 3, 185–187. doi: 10.1080/13697130902973227.

9 Donovitz, G.S. (2022) 'A personal prospective on testosterone therapy in women: What we know in 2022.' *Journal of Personalized Medicine* 12, 8, 1194. doi: 10.3390/jpm12081194.

10 Rivier, C. and Rivest, S. (1991) 'Effect of stress on the activity of the hypothalamic-pituitary-gonadal axis: peripheral and central mechanisms.' *Biol Reprod.* 45, 4, 523–532. doi: 10.1095/biolreprod45.4.523.

11 Bottiglioni, F., de Aloysio, D., Nicoletti, G., Mauloni, M., Mantuano, R. and Capelli, M. (1983) 'A study of thyroid function in the pre- and post-menopause.' *Maturitas* 5, 2, 105–114. doi: 10.1016/0378-5122(83)90006-3.

12 Fanciulli, G., Delitala, A. and Delitala, G. (2009) 'Growth hormone, menopause and ageing: No definite evidence for "rejuvenation" with growth hormone.' *Human Reproduction Update* 15, 3, 341–358. doi: 10.1093/humupd/dmp005.

13 Lizcano, F. and Guzmán, G. (2014) 'Estrogen deficiency and the origin of obesity during menopause.' *BioMed Research International* 2014, 757461. doi: 10.1155/2014/757461.

Chapter 2

1 Baral, S. and Kaphle, H.P. (2023) 'Health-related quality of life among menopausal women: A cross-sectional study from Pokhara, Nepal.' *PLoS One* 18, 1, e0280632. doi: 10.1371/journal.pone.0280632.

2 Monteleone, P., Mascagni, G., Giannini, A., Genazzani, A.R. and Simoncini, T. (2018) 'Symptoms of menopause – global prevalence, physiology and implications.' *Nature Reviews. Endocrinology* 14, 4, 199–215. doi: 10.1038/nrendo.2017.180.

3 Santoro, N., Epperson, C.N. and Mathews, S.B. (2015) 'Menopausal symptoms and their management.' *Endocrinology and Metabolism Clinics of North America* 44, 3, 497–515. doi: 10.1016/j.ecl.2015.05.001.

4 Guthrie, J.R., Dennerstein, L., Taffe, J.R. and Donnelly, V. (2003) 'Heath care-seeking for menopausal problems.' *Climacteric* 6, 2, 112–117. PMID: 12841881.

5 Khunger, N. and Mehrotra, K. (2019) 'Menopausal acne – Challenges and solutions.' *International Journal of Women's Health* 11, 555–567. doi: 10.2147/IJWH.S174292.

6 Lephart, E.D. and Naftolin, F. (2021) 'Menopause and the skin: Old favorites and new innovations in cosmeceuticals for estrogen-deficient skin.' *Dermatology and Therapy (Heidelberg)* 11, 1, 53–69. doi: 10.1007/s13555-020-00468-7.

7 Asserin, J., Lati, E., Shioya, T. and Prawitt, J. (2015) 'The effect of oral collagen peptide supplementation on skin moisture and the dermal collagen network: Evidence from an ex vivo model and randomized, placebo-controlled clinical trials.' *Journal of Cosmetic Dermatology* 14, 4, 291–301. doi: 10.1111/jocd.12174.

8 Proksch, E., Segger, D., Degwert, J., Schunck, M., Zague, V. and Oesser, S. (2014) 'Oral supplementation of specific collagen peptides has beneficial effects on human skin physiology: A double-blind, placebo-controlled study.' *Skin Pharmacology and Physiology* 27, 1, 47–55. doi: 10.1159/000351376.

9 Jenkins, G., Wainwright, L.J., Holland, R., Barrett, K.E. and Casey, J. (2014) 'Wrinkle reduction in post-menopausal women consuming a novel oral supplement: A double-blind placebo-controlled randomized study.' *International Journal of Cosmetic Science* 36, 1, 22–31. doi: 10.1111/ics.12087.

10 Zouboulis, C.C., Blume-Peytavi, U., Kosmadaki, M., Roó, E., *et al.* (2022) 'Skin, hair and beyond: The impact of menopause.' *Climacteric* 25, 5, 434–442. doi: 10.1080/13697137.2022.2050206.

11 Chaikittisilpa, S., Rattanasirisin, N., Panchaprateep, R., Orprayoon, N., *et al.* (2022) 'Prevalence of female pattern hair loss in postmenopausal women: A cross-sectional study.' *Menopause (New York, N.Y.)* 29, 4, 415–420. doi: 10.1097/GME.0000000000001927.

12 Goluch-Koniuszy, Z.S. (2016) 'Nutrition of women with hair loss problem during the period of menopause.' *Przeglad Menopauzalny [Menopause Review]* 15, 1, 56–61. doi: 10.5114/pm.2016.58776.

13 Ghosh, T.S., Shanahan, F. and O'Toole, P.W. (2022) 'The gut microbiome as a modulator of healthy ageing.' *Nature Reviews Gastroenterology & Hepatology* 19, 565–584. https://doi.org/10.1038/s41575-022-00605-x.

14 Peters, B.A., Santoro, N., Kaplan, R.C., Qi, Q. (2022) 'Spotlight on the Gut Microbiome in Menopause: Current Insights.' *Int J Womens Health*, 14, 1059–1072. doi: 10.2147/IJWH.S340491

15 Woudstra, T. and Thomson, A.B. (2002) 'Nutrient absorption and intestinal adaptation with ageing.' *Best Practice & Research. Clinical Gastroenterology* 16, 1, 1–15. doi: 10.1053/bega.2001.0262.

16 Lim, E.Y., Lee, S.Y., Shin, H.S., Lee, J., *et al.* (2020) 'The effect of *Lactobacillus acidophilus* YT1 (MENOLACTO) on improving menopausal symptoms: A randomized, double-blinded, placebo-controlled clinical trial.' *Journal of Clinical Medicine* 9, 7, 2173. doi: 10.3390/jcm9072173.

17 Avis, N.E., Crawford, S.L. and Green, R. (2018) 'Vasomotor symptoms across the menopause transition: Differences among women.' *Obstetrics and Gynecology Clinics of North America* 45, 4, 629–640. doi: 10.1016/j.ogc.2018.07.005.

18 Bansal, R. and Aggarwal, N. (2019) 'Menopausal hot flashes: A concise review.' *Journal of Mid-Life Health* 10, 1, 6–13. doi: 10.4103/jmh.JMH_7_19.

19 Herber-Gast, G.C. and Mishra, G.D. (2013) 'Fruit, Mediterranean-style, and high-fat and -sugar diets are associated with the risk of night sweats and hot flushes in midlife: Results from a prospective cohort study.' *The American Journal of Clinical Nutrition* 97, 5, 1092–1099. doi: 10.3945/ajcn.112.049965.

20 Barnard, N.D., Kahleova, H., Holtz, D.N., Znayenko-Miller, T., *et al.* (2023) 'A dietary intervention for vasomotor symptoms of menopause: A randomized, controlled trial.' *Menopause (New York, N.Y.)* 30, 1, 80–87. doi: 10.1097/GME.0000000000002080.

21 Taku, K., Melby, M.K., Kronenberg, F., Kurzer, M.S. and Messina, M. (2012) 'Extracted or synthesized soybean isoflavones reduce menopausal hot flash frequency and severity: Systematic review and meta-analysis of randomized controlled trials.' *Menopause*, 19, 776–790. doi: 10.1097/gme.0b013e3182410159.

22 Taha, N.H. and Dizaye, K. (2022) 'Impact of *Zingiber officinale* on symptoms and hormonal changes during the menopausal period – A clinical trial in Duhok, Iraq.' *Journal of Natural Science, Biology and Medicine* 13, 2. doi: 10.4103/jnsbm.JNSBM_13_2_7.

23 Borud, E.K., Alraek, T., White, A. *et al.* (2009) 'The Acupuncture on Hot Flushes Among Menopausal Women (ACUFLASH)

study, a randomized controlled trial.' *Menopause* 16, 3, 484–493.

24 Ge, Y., Zhou, S., Li, Y., Wang, Z., *et al.* (2019) 'Estrogen prevents articular cartilage destruction in a mouse model of AMPK deficiency via ERK-mTOR pathway.' *Annals of Translational Medicine* 7, 14, 336. doi: 10.21037/atm.2019.06.77.

25 Purzand, B., Rokhgireh, S., Shabani Zanjani, M., Eshraghi, N., *et al.* (2020) 'The comparison of the effect of soybean and fish oil on supplementation on menopausal symptoms in postmenopausal women: A randomized, double-blind, placebo-controlled trial.' *Complementary Therapies in Clinical Practice* 41, 101239. doi: 10.1016/j.ctcp.2020.101239.

26 Gandhi, J., Chen, A., Dagur, G., Suh, Y., *et al.* (2016) 'Genitourinary syndrome of menopause: An overview of clinical manifestations, pathophysiology, etiology, evaluation, and management.' *American Journal of Obstetrics and Gynecology* 215, 6, 704–711. doi: 10.1016/j.ajog.2016.07.045.

27 Taher, Y.A., Ben Emhemed, H.M. and Tawati, A.M. (2013) 'Menopausal age, related factors and climacteric symptoms in Libyan women.' *Climacteric* 16, 1, 179–184. doi: 10.3109/13697137.2012.682107.

28 Moral, E., Delgado, J.L., Carmona, F., Caballero, B., *et al.*, as the writing group of the GENISSE study (2018) 'Genitourinary syndrome of menopause. Prevalence and quality of life in Spanish postmenopausal women. The GENISSE study.' *Climacteric* 21, 2, 167–173. doi: 10.1080/13697137.2017.1421921.

29 Park, M.G., Cho, S. and Oh, M.M. (2023) 'Menopausal changes in the microbiome: A review focused on the genitourinary microbiome.' *Diagnostics (Basel, Switzerland)* 13, 6, 1193. doi: 10.3390/diagnostics13061193.

30 Goncharenko, V., Bubnov, R., Polivka, J. Jr, Zubor, P., *et al.* (2019) 'Vaginal dryness: Individualised patient profiles, risks and mitigating measures.' *The EPMA Journal* 10, 1, 73–79. doi: 10.1007/s13167-019-00164-3.

31 Larmo, P.S., Yang, B., Hyssälä, J., Kallio, H.P. and Erkkola, R. (2014) 'Effects of sea buckthorn oil intake on vaginal atrophy in postmenopausal women: A randomized, double-blind, placebo-controlled study.' *Maturitas* 79, 3, 316–321. doi: 10.1016/j.maturitas.2014.07.010.

32 Noll, P.R.E.S., Campos, C.A.S., Leone, C., Zangirolami-Raimundo, J., *et al.* (2021) 'Dietary intake and menopausal symptoms in postmenopausal women: A systematic review.' *Climacteric* 24, 2, 128–138. doi: 10.1080/13697137.2020.1828854.

33 Gleason, J.L., Richter, H.E., Redden, D.T., Goode, P.S., Burgio, K.L. and Markland, A.D. (2013) 'Caffeine and urinary incontinence in US women.' *International Urogynecology Journal* 24, 2, 295–302. doi: 10.1007/s00192-012-1829-5.

Part 2

1 McCarthy, M. and Raval, A.P. (2020) 'The peri-menopause in a woman's life: A systemic inflammatory phase that enables later neurodegenerative disease.' *Journal of Neuroinflammation* 17, 317. https://doi.org/10.1186/s12974-020-01998-9

2 Sternberg, E.M. (2001) 'Neuroendocrine regulation of autoimmune/inflammatory disease.' *The Journal of Endocrinology* 169, 3, 429–435. doi: 10.1677/joe.0.1690429.

3 Girasole, G., Giuliani, N., Modena, A.B., Passeri, G. and Pedrazzoni, M. (1999) 'Oestrogens prevent the increase of human serum soluble interleukin-6 receptor induced by ovariectomy in vivo and decrease its release in human osteoblastic cells in vitro.' *Clinical Endocrinology* 51, 6, 801–807. doi: 10.1046/j.1365-2265.1999.00896.x.

4 Yasui, T., Maegawa, M., Tomita, J., Miyatani, Y., et al. (2007) 'Changes in serum cytokine concentrations during the menopausal transition.' *Maturitas* 56, 4, 396–403. doi: 10.1016/j.maturitas.2006.11.002.

Chapter 3

1 Erdélyi, A., Pálfi, E., Tűű, L. *et al.* (2023) 'The Importance of Nutrition in Menopause and Perimenopause-A Review.' *Nutrients* 16, 1, 27. doi: 10.3390/nu16010027.

2 Lurati, A.R. (2018) 'Effects of menopause on appetite and the gastrointestinal system.' *Nursing for Women's Health* 22, 6, 499–505. https://doi.org/10.1016/j.nwh.2018.09.004.

3 Ma, R., Mikhail, M.E., Culbert, K.M., Johnson, A.W., Sisk, C.L. and Klump, K.L. (2020) 'Ovarian hormones and reward processes in palatable food intake and binge eating.' *Physiology (Bethesda)* 35, 1, 69–78. doi: 10.1152/physiol.00013.2019.

4 Sharma, S. and Kavuru, M. (2010) 'Sleep and metabolism: An overview.' *International Journal of Endocrinology* 2010, 270832. doi: 10.1155/2010/270832.

5 Rettberg, J.R., Yao, J. and Brinton, R.D. (2014) 'Estrogen: A master regulator of bioenergetic systems in the brain and body.'

Frontiers in Neuroendocrinology 35, 1, 8–30. doi: 10.1016/j.yfrne.2013.08.001.

6 Poehlman, E.T. (2002) 'Menopause, energy expenditure, and body composition.' *Acta Obstet. Gynecol. Scand.*, 81, 603–611. doi: 10.1034/j.1600-0412.2002.810705.x.

7 Bottiglioni, F., de Aloysio, D., Nicoletti, G., Mauloni, M., Mantuano, R., Capelli, M. (1983) 'A study of thyroid function in the pre- and post-menopause.' *Maturitas* 5, 2, 105–114. doi: 10.1016/0378-5122(83)90006-3.

8 Hyvärinen, M., Juppi, H.K., Taskinen, S., Karppinen, J.E., *et al.* (2022) 'Metabolic health, menopause, and physical activity: A 4-year follow-up study.' *International Journal of Obesity (London)* 46, 3, 544–554. doi: 10.1038/s41366-021-01022-x.

9 Volpi, E., Nazemi, R. and Fujita, S. (2004) 'Muscle tissue changes with aging.' *Current Opinion in Clinical Nutrition and Metabolic Care* 7, 4, 405–410. doi: 10.1097/01.mco.0000134362.76653.b2.

10 Sternfeld, B., Bhat, A.K., Wang, H., Sharp, T. and Quesenberry Jr, C.P. (2005) 'Menopause, physical activity, and body composition/fat distribution in midlife women.' *Medicine and Science in Sports and Exercise* 37, 7, 1195–1202. doi: 10.1249/01.mss.0000170083.41186.b1.

11 Leidy, H.J., Ortinau, L.C., Douglas, S.M. and Hoertel, H.A. (2013) 'Beneficial effects of a higher-protein breakfast on the appetitive, hormonal, and neural signals controlling energy intake regulation in overweight/obese, "breakfast-skipping," late-adolescent girls.' *The American Journal of Clinical Nutrition* 97, 4, 677–688. doi: 10.3945/ajcn.112.053116.

12 Perraudeau, F., McMurdie, P., Bullard, J., Cheng, A. *et al.* (2020) 'Improvements to postprandial glucose control in subjects with type 2 diabetes: A multicenter, double blind, randomized placebo-controlled trial of a novel probiotic formulation.' *BMJ Open Diabetes Research & Care* 8, 1, e001319. doi: 10.1136/bmjdrc-2020-001319.

13 Depommier, C., Everard, A., Druart, C., Plovier, H., *et al.* (2019) 'Supplementation with *Akkermansia muciniphila* in overweight and obese human volunteers: A proof-of-concept exploratory study.' *Nature Medicine* 25, 7, 1096–1103. doi: 10.1038/s41591-019-0495-2.

14 Bellini, A., Nicolò, A., Bazzucchi, I. and Sacchetti, M. (2022) 'The effects of postprandial walking on the glucose response after meals with different characteristics.' *Nutrients* 14, 5, 1080. doi: 10.3390/nu14051080.

15 Baskaran, K., Ahamath, B.K., Shanmugasundaram, K.R. and Shanmugasundaram, E.R.

(1990) 'Antidiabetic effect of a leaf extract from *Gymnema sylvestre* in non-insulin-dependent diabetes mellitus patients.' *Journal of Ethnopharmacology* 30, 3, 295–300. doi: 10.1016/0378-8741(90)90108-6.

16 Rochlani, Y., Pothineni, N.V., Kovelamudi, S. and Mehta, J.L. (2017) 'Metabolic syndrome: Pathophysiology, management, and modulation by natural compounds.' *Therapeutic Advances in Cardiovascular Disease* 11, 8, 215–225. doi: 10.1177/1753944717711379.

17 Leung, L., Birtwhistle, R., Kotecha, J., Hannah, S. and Cuthbertson, S. (2009) 'Anti-diabetic and hypoglycaemic effects of *Momordica charantia* (bitter melon): A mini review.' *The British Journal of Nutrition* 102, 12, 1703–1708. doi: 10.1017/S0007114509992054.

18 Kamenova, P. (2006) 'Improvement of insulin sensitivity in patients with type 2 diabetes mellitus after oral administration of alpha-lipoic acid.' *Hormones (Athens, Greece)* 5, 4, 251–258. doi: 10.14310/horm.2002.11191.

19 Koh, E.H., Lee, W.J., Lee, S.A., Kim, E.H. *et al.* (2011) 'Effects of alpha-lipoic acid on body weight in obese subjects.' *The American Journal of Medicine* 124, 1, 85.e1–8. doi: 10.1016/j.amjmed.2010.08.005.

20 Ghelani, H., Razmovski-Naumovski, V. and Nammi, S. (2017) 'Chronic treatment of (R)-α-lipoic acid reduces blood glucose and lipid levels in high-fat diet and low-dose streptozotocin-induced metabolic syndrome and type 2 diabetes in Sprague-Dawley rats.' *Pharmacology Research & Perspectives* 5, 3, e00306. doi: 10.1002/prp2.306.

21 Koh, E.H., Lee, W.J., Lee, S.A., Kim, E.H. *et al.* (2011) 'Effects of alpha-lipoic acid on body weight in obese subjects.' *The American Journal of Medicine* 124, 1, 85.e1–8. doi: 10.1016/j.amjmed.2010.08.005.

22 Yin, J., Xing, H. and Ye, J. (2008) 'Efficacy of berberine in patients with type 2 diabetes mellitus.' *Metabolism* 57, 5, 712–717. doi: 10.1016/j.metabol.2008.01.013.

23 Han, Y., Xiang, Y., Shi, Y., Tang. X., *et al.* (2021) 'Pharmacokinetics and pharmacological activities of berberine in diabetes mellitus treatment.' *Evidence-Based Complementary and Alternative Medicine* 2021, 9987097. doi: 10.1155/2021/9987097.

24 Cicero, A.F. and Baggioni, A. (2016) 'Berberine and its role in chronic disease.' *Advances in Experimental Medicine and Biology* 928, 27–45. doi: 10.1007/978-3-319-41334-1_2.

25 Anderson, R.A., Polansky, M.M., Bryden, N.A., Bhathena, S.J. and Canary, J.J. (1987) 'Effects of supplemental chromium on patients with symptoms of

reactive hypoglycemia.' *Metabolism: Clinical and Experimental* 36, 4, 351–355. doi: 10.1016/0026-0495(87)90206-x.

26 Albarracin, C.A., Fuqua, B.C., Evans, J.L. and Goldfine, I.D. (2008) 'Chromium picolinate and biotin combination improves glucose metabolism in treated, uncontrolled overweight to obese patients with type 2 diabetes.' *Diabetes/Metabolism Research and Reviews* 24, 1, 41–51. doi: 10.1002/dmrr.755.

27 Paiva, A.N., de Lima, J.G., de Medeiros, A.C.Q., Figueiredo, H.A.O., *et al.* (2015) 'Beneficial effects of oral chromium picolinate supplementation on glycemic control in patients with type 2 diabetes: A rand-omized clinical study.' *Journal of Trace Elements in Medicine and Biology* 32, 66–72. doi: 10.1016/j.jtemb.2015.05.006.

28 Willoughby, D., Hewlings, S. and Kalman, D. (2018) 'Body composition changes in weight loss: Strategies and supplementation for maintaining lean body mass, a brief review.' *Nutrients* 10, 12, 1876. doi: 10.3390/nu10121876.

29 Fuhr Jr, J.P., He, H., Goldfarb, N. and Nash, D.B. (2005) 'Use of chromium picolinate and biotin in the management of type 2 diabetes: An economic analysis.' *Disease Management* 8, 4, 265–275. doi: 10.1089/dis.2005.8.265.

Chapter 4

1 Ryczkowska, K., Adach, W., Janikowski, K., Banach, M. and Bielecka-Dabrowa, A. (2022) 'Menopause and women's cardiovascular health: Is it really an obvious relationship?' *Archives of Medical Science* 19, 2, 458–466. doi: 10.5114/aoms/157308.

2 Katerina, S. and Alevizaki, M. (2007) 'Coronary heart disease in postmenopausal women; the role of endogenous estrogens and their receptors.' *Hormones* 6, 1, 9–24.

3 Mauvais-Jarvis, F., Clegg, D.J. and Hevener, A.L. (2013) 'The role of estrogens in control of energy balance and glucose homeostasis.' *Endocrine Reviews* 34, 3, 309–338. doi: 10.1210/er.2012-1055.

4 Ko, S.-H. and Kim, H.-S. (2020) 'Menopause-associated lipid metabolic disorders and foods beneficial for postmenopausal women.' *Nutrients* 12, 1, 202. doi: 10.3390/nu12010202.

5 Matthews, K.A., Crawford, S.L., Chae, C.U., *et al.* (2009) 'Are changes in cardiovascular disease risk factors in midlife women due to chronological aging or to the menopausal transition?' *J Am Coll Cardiol*, 54, 25, 2366–2373. doi: 10.1016/j.jacc.2009.10.009.

6 Gersh, F.L., O'Keefe, J.H., Lavie, C.J. and Henry, B.M. (2021) 'The renin-angiotensin-aldosterone system in postmenopausal women: The promise of hormone therapy.' *Mayo Clinic Proceedings* 96, 12, 3130–3141. doi: 10.1016/j.mayocp.2021.08.009.

7 Chakrabarti, S., Lekontseva, O. and Davidge, S.T. (2008) 'Estrogen is a modulator of vascular inflammation.' *IUBMB Life*, 60, 6, 376–382. doi: 10.1002/iub.48.

8 Iorga, A., Cunningham, C.M., Moazeni, S., Ruffenach, G., Umar, S. and Eghbali, M. (2017) 'The protective role of estrogen and estrogen receptors in cardiovascular disease and the controversial use of estrogen therapy.' *Biology of Sex Differences* 8, 1, 33. doi: 10.1186/s13293-017-0152-8.

9 Gersh, F.L., O'Keefe, J.H., Lavie, C.J. and Henry, B.M. (2021) 'The renin-angiotensin-aldosterone system in postmenopausal women: The promise of hormone therapy.' *Mayo Clinic Proceedings* 96, 12, 3130–3141. doi: 10.1016/j.mayocp.2021.08.009.

10 Mauvais-Jarvis, F., Clegg, D.J. and Hevener, A.L. (2013) 'The role of estrogens in control of energy balance and glucose homeostasis.' *Endocrine Reviews* 34, 3, 309–338. doi: 10.1210/er.2012-1055.

11 Nevzati, E., Shafighi, M., Bakhtian, K.D., Treiber, H., Fandino, J., Fathi, A.R. (2015) 'Estrogen induces nitric oxide production via nitric oxide synthase activation in endothelial cells.' *Acta Neurochir Suppl.*, 120, 141–145. doi: 10.1007/978-3-319-04981-6_24.

12 Yang, X.-P. and Reckelhoff, J.F. (2011) 'Estrogen, hormonal replacement therapy and cardiovascular disease.' *Current Opinion in Nephrology and Hypertension* 20, 2, 133–138. doi: 10.1097/MNH.0b013e3283431921.

13 Lei, L., Zhao, N., Zhang, L., Chen, J., Lu, X. and Piao, S. (2022) 'Gut microbiota is a potential goalkeeper of dyslipidemia.' *Frontiers in Endocrinology (Lausanne)* 13, 950826. doi: 10.3389/fendo.2022.950826.

14 Peters, B.A., Santoro, N., Kaplan, R.C. and Qi, Q. (2022) 'Spotlight on the gut microbiome in menopause: Current insights.' *International Journal of Women's Health* 14, 1059–1072. doi: 10.2147/IJWH.S340491.

15 Wu, H. and Chiou, J. (2021) 'Potential benefits of probiotics and prebiotics for coronary heart disease and stroke.' *Nutrients* 13, 8, 2878. doi: 10.3390/nu13082878.

16 Avery, E.G., Bartolomaeus, H., Maifeld, A., Marko, L., *et al.* (2021) 'The gut microbiome in hypertension: Recent advances and future perspectives.' *Circulation Research* 128, 7, 934–950. doi: 10.1161/CIRCRESAHA.121.318065.

17 Simon, M.C., Strassburger, K., Nowotny, B., Kolb, H., *et al.* (2015) 'Intake of *Lactobacillus reuteri* improves incretin and insulin secretion in glucose-tolerant humans: A proof of concept.' *Diabetes Care 38*, 10, 1827–1834. doi: 10.2337/dc14-2690.

18 Park, Y., Subar, A.F., Hollenbeck, A. and Schatzkin, A. (2011) 'Dietary fiber intake and mortality in the NIH-AARP diet and health study.' *Archives of Internal Medicine 171*, 12, 1061–1068. doi: 10.1001/archinternmed.2011.18.

19 Bihuniak, J.D., Ramos, A., Huedo-Medina, T., Hutchins-Wiese, H., Kerstetter, J.E. and Kenny, A.M. (2016) 'Adherence to a Mediterranean-style diet and its influence on cardiovascular risk factors in postmenopausal women.' *Journal of the Academy of Nutrition and Dietetics 116*, 11, 1767–1775. doi: 10.1016/j.jand.2016.06.377.

20 Mendoza, K., Smith-Warner, S.A., Rossato, S.L. *et al.* (2024) 'Ultra-processed foods and cardiovascular disease: analysis of three large US prospective cohorts and a systematic review and meta-analysis of prospective cohort studies.' Lancet Reg Health Am., 37, 100859. doi: 10.1016/j.lana.2024.100859.

21 Wang, H.-P., Yang, J., Qin, L.-Q. and Yang, X.-J. (2015) 'Effect of garlic on blood pressure: A meta-analysis.' *The Journal of Clinical Hypertension (Greenwich)* 17, 3, 223–231. doi: 10.1111/jch.12473; Ried, K., Toben, C. and Fakler, P. (2013) 'Effect of garlic on serum lipids: An updated meta-analysis.' *Nutrition Reviews 71*, 5, 282–299. doi: 10.1111/nure.12012.

22 Wolters, M., Dejanovic, G.M., Asllanaj, E., Günther, K., et al. (2020) 'Effects of phytoestrogen supplementation on intermediate cardiovascular disease risk factors among postmenopausal women: A meta-analysis of randomized controlled trials.' *Menopause (New York, NY) 27*, 9, 1081–1092. doi: 10.1097/GME.0000000000001566.

23 Yamagata, K. (2019) 'Polyphenols regulate endothelial functions and reduce the risk of cardiovascular disease.' *Current Pharmaceutical Design 25*, 22, 2443–2458. doi: 10.2174/1381612825666190722100504.

24 Pinaffi-Langley, A.C., Dajani, R.M., Prater, M.C. *et al.* (2025) 'Dietary Nitrate from Plant Foods: A Conditionally Essential Nutrient for Cardiovascular Health' *Advances in Nutrition, 15*, 1, 100158.

25 Machha, A. and Schechter, A.N. (2011) 'Dietary nitrite and nitrate: A review of potential mechanisms of cardiovascular benefits.' *European Journal of Nutrition 50*, 5, 293–303. doi: 10.1007/s00394-011-0192-5.

Chapter 5

1 Scott, E.L., Zhang, Q.G., Vadlamudi, R.K. and Brann, D.W. (2014) 'Premature menopause and risk of neurological disease: Basic mechanisms and clinical implications.' *Molecular and Cellular Endocrinology 389*, 1–2, 2–6. doi: 10.1016/j.mce.2014.01.013.

2 Ooishi, Y., Kawato, S., Hojo, Y., Hatanaka, Y., *et al.* (2012) 'Modulation of synaptic plasticity in the hippocampus by hippocampus-derived estrogen and androgen.' *The Journal of Steroid Biochemistry and Molecular Biology 131*, 1–2, 37–51. doi: 10.1016/j.jsbmb.2011.10.004.

3 Hojo, Y., Higo, S., Kawato, S., Hatanaka, Y., *et al.* (2011) 'Hippocampal synthesis of sex steroids and corticosteroids: Essential for modulation of synaptic plasticity.' *Frontiers in Endocrinology (Lausanne) 2*, 43. doi: 10.3389/fendo.2011.00043.

4 Toffol, E., Heikinheimo, O. and Partonen, T. (2013) 'Associations between psychological well-being, mental health, and hormone therapy in perimenopausal and postmenopausal women: Results of two population-based studies.' *Menopause (New York, N.Y.) 20*, 6, 667–676, doi: 10.1097/gme.0b013e318278eec1.

5 Rettberg, J.R., Yao, J. and Diaz Brinton, R. (2014) 'Estrogen: A master regulator of bioenergetic systems in the brain and body.' *Frontiers in Neuroendocrinology 35*, 1, 8–30. doi: 10.1016/j.yfrne.2013.08.001.

6 Chakrabarti, S., Munshi, S., Banerjee, K., Thakurta, I.G., Sinha, M. and Bagh, M.B. (2011) 'Mitochondrial dysfunction during brain aging: Role of oxidative stress and modulation by antioxidant supplementation.' *Aging and Disease 2*, 3, 242–256. PMID: 22396876.

7 Scott, E., Zhang, Q.G., Wang, R., Vadlamudi, R. and Brann, D. (2012) 'Estrogen neuroprotection and the critical period hypothesis.' *Frontiers in Neuroendocrinology 33*, 1, 85–104. doi: 10.1016/j.yfrne.2011.10.001.

8 Scott, E., Zhang, Q.G., Wang, R., Vadlamudi, R. and Brann, D. (2012) 'Estrogen neuroprotection and the critical period hypothesis.' *Frontiers in Neuroendocrinology 33*, 1, 85–104. doi: 10.1016/j.yfrne.2011.10.001.

9 Mosconi, L., Berti, V., Quinn, C., McHugh, P., *et al.* (2017) 'Perimenopause and emergence of an Alzheimer's bioenergetic phenotype in brain and periphery.' *PLoS ONE 12*, 10, e0185926. doi: 10.1371/journal.pone.0185926.

10 Paganini-Hill, A. and Henderson, V.W. (1994) 'Estrogen deficiency and risk of Alzheimer's disease in women.' *American Journal of Epidemiology* 140, 3, 256–261. doi: 10.1093/oxfordjournals.aje.a117244.

11 Jacobs, E.G., Weiss, B.K., Makris, N., Whitfield-Gabrieli, W., *et al.* (2016) 'Impact of sex and menopausal status on episodic memory circuitry in early midlife.' *The Journal of Neuroscience* 36, 39, 10163–10173. doi: 10.1523/JNEUROSCI.0951-16.2016.

12 Tayebati, S.K., Tomassoni, D., Di Stefano, A., Sozio, P. and Amenta, F. (2009) 'Influence of treatment with CDP-choline or choline alphoscerate on brain dopamine and acetylcholine transporters.' *Journal of the Neurological Sciences* 283, 1–2, 285.

13 Balter, L.J., Bosch, J.A., Aldred, S., Drayson, M.T., *et al.* (2019) 'Selective effects of acute low-grade inflammation on human visual attention.' *Neuroimage* 202, 116098. doi: 10.1016/j.neuroimage.2019.116098.

14 Stachenfeld, N.S. (2014) 'Hormonal changes during menopause and the impact on fluid regulation.' *Reprod Sci.* 21, 5, 555–561. doi: 10.1177/1933719113518992.

15 Bromberger, J.T. and Epperson, C.N. (2018) 'Depression during and after the perimenopause: Impact of hormones, genetics, and environmental determinants of disease.' *Obstetrics and Gynecology Clinics of North America* 45, 4, 663–678. doi: 10.1016/j.ogc.2018.07.007.

16 Almey, A., Milner, T.A. and Brake, W.G. (2015) 'Estrogen receptors in the central nervous system and their implication for dopamine-dependent cognition in females.' *Hormones and Behavior* 74, 125–138. doi: 10.1016/j.yhbeh.2015.06.010.

17 Rybaczyk, L.A., Bashaw, M.J., Pathak, D.R., Moody, S.M., Gilders, R.M. and Holzschu, D.L. (2005) 'An overlooked connection: Serotonergic mediation of estrogen-related physiology and pathology.' *BMC Women's Health* 5, 12. doi: 10.1186/1472-6874-5-12.

18 Pearlstein, T., Rosen, K. and Stone, A.B. (1997) 'Mood disorders and menopause.' *Endocrinology and Metabolism Clinics of North America* 26, 2, 279–294. doi: 10.1016/s0889-8529(05)70247-4.

19 Li, Q.Q., Shi, G.X., Xu, Q., Wang, J., Liu, C.Z. and Wang, L.P. (2013) 'Acupuncture effect and central autonomic regulation.' *Evidence-Based Complementary and Alternative Medicine* 2013, 267959. doi: 10.1155/2013/267959.

20 Singh, M,. Su, C. (2013) 'Progesterone-induced neuroprotection: factors that may predict therapeutic efficacy.' *Brain Res.* 1514, 98–106. doi: 10.1016/j.brainres.2013.01.027.

21 Standeven, L.R., McEvoy, K.O. and Osborne, L.M. (2020) 'Progesterone, reproduction, and psychiatric illness.' *Best Pract Res Clin Obstet Gynaecol* 69, 108–126. doi: 10.1016/j.bpobgyn.2020.06.001.

22 Maharjan, D.T., Syed, A.A.S., Lin, G.N. and Ying, W. (2021) 'Testosterone in female depression: A meta-analysis and mendelian randomization study.' *Biomolecules* 11, 3, 409. doi: 10.3390/biom11030409.

23 Durdiakova, J., Ostatnikova, D. and Celec, P. (2011) 'Testosterone and its metabolites – Modulators of brain functions.' *Acta Neurobiologiae Experimentalis* 71, 4, 434–454. doi: 10.55782/ane-2011-1863.

24 Celec, P., Ostatníková, D. and Hodosy, J. (2015) 'On the effects of testosterone on brain behavioral functions.' *Frontiers in Neuroscience* 9, 12. doi: 10.3389/fnins.2015.00012.

25 Dodd, G.F., Williams, C.M., Butler, L.T. and Spencer, J.P.E. (2019) 'Acute effects of flavonoid-rich blueberry on cognitive and vascular function in healthy older adults.' *Nutrition and Healthy Aging* 5, 2, 119–132. doi:10.3233/NHA-180056.

26 Karsten, H.D., Patterson, P.H., Stout, R. and Crews, G. (2010) 'Vitamins A, E and fatty acid composition of the eggs of caged hens and pastured hens.' *Renewable Agriculture and Food Systems* 25, 1, 45–54. doi: 10.1017/S1742170509990214.

27 Jang, C.H., Oh, J., Lim, J.S., Kim, H.J. and Kim, J.S. (2021) 'Fermented soy products: Beneficial potential in neurodegenerative diseases.' *Foods (Basel, Switzerland)* 10, 3, 636. doi: 10.3390/foods10030636.

28 Foshati, S., Ghanizadeh, A. and Akhlaghi, M. (2022) 'Extra-virgin olive oil improves depression symptoms without affecting salivary cortisol and brain-derived neurotrophic factor in patients with major depression: A double-blind randomized controlled trial.' *Journal of the Academy of Nutrition and Dietetics* 122, 2, 284–297.e1. doi: 10.1016/j.jand.2021.07.016.

29 Jiang, C., Sakakibara, E., Lin, W.J., Wang, J., Pasinetti, G.M. and Salton, S.R. (2019) 'Grape-derived polyphenols produce antidepressant effects via VGF- and BDNF-dependent mechanisms.' *Annals of the New York Academy of Sciences* 1455, 1, 196–205. doi: 10.1111/nyas.14098.

30 Surendran, G., Saye, J., Binti Mohd Jalil, S. *et al.* (2025) 'Acute effects of a standardised extract of Hericium erinaceus (Lion's Mane mushroom) on cognition and mood in healthy younger adults: a double-blind randomised placebo-controlled study.' *Front Nutr.* 12, 1405796. doi: 10.3389/fnut.2025.1405796.

Chapter 6

1 Ginaldi, L., Di Benedetto, M.C. and De Martinis, M. (2005) 'Osteoporosis, inflammation and ageing.' *Immunity & Ageing* 2, 14. doi: 10.1186/1742-4933-2-14.

2 Swanson, C.M., Kohrt, W.M., Buxton, O.M., Everson, C.A., *et al.* (2018) 'The importance of the circadian system & sleep for bone health.' *Metabolism: Clinical and Experimental 84*, 28–43. doi: 10.1016/j.metabol.2017.12.002.

3 Ochs-Balcom, H.M., Hovey, K.M., Andrews, C., Cauley, J.A., *et al.* (2020) 'Short sleep is associated with low bone mineral density and osteoporosis in the women's health initiative.' *Journal of Bone and Mineral Research 35*, 2, 261–268. doi: 10.1002/jbmr.3879.

4 Vainionpää, A., Korpelainen, R., Leppäluoto, J. and Jämsä, T. (2005) 'Effects of high-impact exercise on bone mineral density: A randomized controlled trial in premenopausal women.' *Osteoporosis International 16*, 2, 191–197. doi: 10.1007/s00198-004-1659-5.

5 Zehnacker, C.H. and Bemis-Dougherty, A. (2007) 'Effect of weighted exercises on bone mineral density in post menopausal women. A systematic review.' *Journal of Geriatric Physical Therapy 30*, 2, 79–88. doi: 10.1519/00139143-200708000-00007.

6 Benedetti, M.G., Furlini, G., Zati, A. and Mauro, G.L. (2018) 'The effectiveness of physical exercise on bone density in osteoporotic patients.' *BioMed Research International 2018*, 4840531. doi: 10.1155/2018/4840531.

7 Daly, R.M., Dalla Via, J., Duckham, R.L., Fraser, S.F. and Helge, E.W. (2019) 'Exercise for the prevention of osteoporosis in postmenopausal women: An evidence-based guide to the optimal prescription.' *Brazilian Journal of Physical Therapy 23*, 2, 170–180. doi: 10.1016/j.bjpt.2018.11.011.

8 Daly, R.M., Dalla Via, J., Duckham, R.L., Fraser, S.F. and Helge, E.W. (2019) 'Exercise for the prevention of osteoporosis in postmenopausal women: An evidence-based guide to the optimal prescription.' *Brazilian Journal of Physical Therapy 23*, 2, 170–180. doi: 10.1016/j.bjpt.2018.11.011.

9 Zdzieblik, D., Oesser, S. and König, D. (2021) 'Specific bioactive collagen peptides in osteopenia and osteoporosis: Long-term observation in postmenopausal women.' *Journal of Bone Metabolism 28*, 3, 207–213. doi: 10.11005/jbm.2021.28.3.207.

10 König, D. and Oesser, S. (2016) 'Report on the study "Impact of specific bioactive collagen peptides (FORTIBONE®) on the bone mineral density in postmenopausal women".' 5 October.

11 Wallace, T.C. (2019) 'Optimizing dietary protein for lifelong bone health: A paradox unraveled.' *Nutrition Today 54*, 3, 107–115. doi: 10.1097/NT.0000000000000340.

12 Mangano, K.M., Sahni, S. and Kerstetter, J.E. (2014) 'Dietary protein is beneficial to bone health under conditions of adequate calcium intake: An update on clinical research.' *Current Opinion in Clinical Nutrition and Metabolic Care 17*, 1, 69–74. doi: 10.1097/MCO.0000000000000013.

13 Management of osteoporosis in postmenopausal women: The 2021 position statement of The North American Menopause Society. (2021) *Menopause*, 28, 973–997. doi: 10.1097/GME.0000000000001831.

14 Wang, K. (2024) 'The potential therapeutic role of curcumin in osteoporosis treatment: Based on multiple signaling pathways.' *Frontiers in Pharmacology 15*, 1446536. doi: 10.3389/fphar.2024.1446536.

Chapter 7

1 Dąbrowska-Galas, M., Dąbrowska, J., Ptaszkowski, K. and Plinta, R. (2019) 'High physical activity level may reduce menopausal symptoms.' *Medicina (Kaunas) 55*, 8, 466. doi: 10.3390/medicina55080466.

2 Zhang, H., Tong, T.K., Qiu, W., Zhang, X., Zhou, S., Liu, Y. and He, Y. (2017) 'Comparable effects of high-intensity interval training and prolonged continuous exercise training on abdominal visceral fat reduction in obese young women.' *Journal of Diabetes Research 2017*, 5071740. doi: 10.1155/2017/5071740.

3 Volpi, E., Nazemi, R. and Fujita, S. (2004) 'Muscle tissue changes with aging.' *Current Opinion in Clinical Nutrition and Metabolic Care 7*, 4, 405–410. doi: 10.1097/01.mco.0000134362.76653.b2.

4 Gregory, G.J., Zepeda, C.S. and Sundberg, C.W. (2022) 'Single muscle fibre contractile function with ageing.' *The Journal of Physiology 600*, 23, 5005–5026. doi: 10.1113/JP282298.

5 Isenmann, E., Kaluza, D., Havers, T., Elbeshausen, A., *et al.* (2023) 'Resistance training alters body composition in middle-aged women depending on menopause – A 20-week control trial.' *BMC Women's Health 23*, 1, 526. doi: 10.1186/s12905-023-02671-y.

6 Lee, H., Caguicla, J.M., Park, S., Kwak, D.J., *et al.* (2016) 'Effects of 8-week Pilates exercise program on menopausal symptoms

and lumbar strength and flexibility in postmenopausal women.' *Journal of Exercise Rehabilitation* 12, 3, 247–251. doi: 10.12965/jer.1632630.315.

7 Smith-Ryan, A.E., Cabre, H.E., Eckerson, J.M. and Candow, D.G. (2021) 'Creatine supplementation in women's health: A lifespan perspective.' *Nutrients* 13, 3, 877. doi: 10.3390/nu13030877.

8 Candow, D.G., Forbes, S.C., Chilibeck, P.D., Cornish, S.M., Antonio, J. and Kreider, R.B. (2019) 'Effectiveness of creatine supplementation on aging muscle and bone: Focus on falls prevention and inflammation.' *Journal of Clinical Medicine* 8, 4, 488. doi: 10.3390/jcm8040488.

9 Chilibeck, P.D., Candow, D.G., Landeryou, T., Kaviani, M. and Paus-Jenssen, L. (2015) 'Effects of creatine and resistance training on bone health in postmenopausal women.' *Medicine and Science in Sports and Exercise* 47, 8, 1587–1595. doi: 10.1249/MSS.0000000000000571.

Chapter 8

1 Hsu, H.C. and Lin, M.H. (2005) 'Exploring quality of sleep and its related factors among menopausal women.' *The Journal of Nursing Research* 13, 2, 153–164. doi: 10.1097/01.jnr.0000387536.60760.4e.

2 Tandon, V.R., Sharma, S., Mahajan, A., Mahajan, A. and Tandon, A. (2022) 'Menopause and sleep disorders.' *Journal of Mid-Life Health* 13, 1, 26–33. doi: 10.4103/jmh.jmh_18_22.

3 Figueiro, M., Plitnick, B. and Rea, M. (2012) 'Light modulates leptin and ghrelin in sleep-restricted adults.' *International Journal of Endocrinology* 2012, 530726. doi: 10.1155/2012/530726.

4 Regestein, Q.R. (1994) 'Menopausal Aspects of Sleep Disturbance.' In J. Lorrain, L. Plouffe, V.A. Ravnikar, L. Speroff and N.B. Watts (eds) *Comprehensive Management of Menopause* (pp.358–366). New York: Springer. https://doi.org/10.1007/978-1-4612-4330-4_34

5 Santhi, N., Lazar, A.S., McCabe, P.J., Lo, J.C., Groeger, J.A. and Dijk, D.J. (2016) 'Sex differences in the circadian regulation of sleep and waking cognition in humans.' *Proceedings of the National Academy of Sciences of the United States of America* 113, 19, E2730–E2739. doi: 10.1073/pnas.1521637113.

6 Kruijver, F.P. and Swaab, D.F. (2002) 'Sex hormone receptors are present in the human suprachiasmatic nucleus.' *Neuroendocrinology* 75, 5, 296–305. doi: 10.1159/000057339.

7 Jehan, S., Giardin, J.-L., Zizi, F., Auguste, E., *et al.* (2017) 'Sleep, melatonin, and the menopausal transition: What are the links?' *Sleep Science* 10, 1, 11–18. doi: 10.5935/1984-0063.20170003.

8 Reid, K.J., Santostasi, G., Baron, K.G., Wilson, J., Kang, J. and Zee, P.C. (2014) 'Timing and intensity of light correlate with body weight in adults.' *PLoS One* 9, 4, e92251. doi: 10.1371/journal.pone.0092251; Cheung, I.N., Zee, P.C., Shalman, D., Malkani, R.G., Kang, J. and Reid, K.J. (2016) 'Morning and evening blue-enriched light exposure alters metabolic function in normal weight adults.' *PLoS One* 11, 5, e0155601. doi: 10.1371/journal.pone.0155601.

9 McMullan, C., Schernhammer, E., Rimm, E., Hu, F. and Forman, J. (2013) 'Melatonin secretion and the incidence of type 2 diabetes.' *JAMA* 309, 13, 1388–1396. doi: 10.1001/jama.2013.2710.

10 Peuhkuri, K., Sihvola, N. and Korpela, R. (2012) 'Dietary factors and fluctuating levels of melatonin.' *Food & Nutrition Research* 56. doi: 10.3402/fnr.v56i0.17252.

11 Garland, S.N., Xie, S.X., DuHamel, K., Bao, T., *et al.* (2019) 'Acupuncture versus cognitive behavioral therapy for insomnia in cancer survivors: A randomized clinical trial. *Journal of the National Cancer Institute* 111, 12, 1323–1331. doi: 10.1093/jnci/djz050.

12 Pigeon, W.R., Carr, M., Gorman, C. and Perlis, M.L. (2010) 'Effects of a tart cherry juice beverage on the sleep of older adults with insomnia: A pilot study.' *Journal of Medicinal Food* 13, 3, 579–583. doi: 10.1089/jmf.2009.0096.

Chapter 9

1 Oliveira, J.F., Dias, N.S., Correia, M. *et al.* (2013) 'Chronic stress disrupts neural coherence between cortico-limbic structures.' *Front Neural Circuits* 7, 10. doi: 10.3389/fncir.2013.00010.

2 Yan, Y.X., Xiao, H.B., Wang, S.S. *et al.* (2016) 'Investigation of the Relationship Between Chronic Stress and Insulin Resistance in a Chinese Population.' *J Epidemiol.* 26, 7, 355–360. doi: 10.2188/jea.JE20150183.

3 Gibson, C.J., Thurston, R.C. and Matthews, K.A. (2016) 'Cortisol dysregulation is associated with daily diary-reported hot flashes among midlife women.' *Clinical Endocrinology* 85, 4, 645–651. https://doi.org/10.1111/cen.13076

4 Reed, S.D., Newton, K.M., Larson, J.C., Booth-LaForce, C. (2016) 'Daily salivary cortisol patterns in midlife women with hot flashes.' *Clinical Endocrinology (Oxford) 84*, 5, 672–679. doi: 10.1111/cen.12995.

5 Randolph, Jr, J.F., Sowers, M.F., Bond-arenko, I., Gold, E.B., *et al.* (2005) 'The relationship of longitudinal change in reproductive hormones and vasomotor symptoms during the menopausal transition.' *The Journal of Clinical Endocrinology & Metabolism 90*, 11, 6106–6112. https://doi.org/10.1210/jc.2005-1374

6 Cagnacci, A., Xholli, A., Fontanesi, F., Neri, I., Facchinetti, F. and Palma, F. (2021) 'Treatment of menopausal symptoms: Concomitant modification of cortisol.' *Menopause (New York, N.Y.) 29*, 1, 23–27. doi: 10.1097/GME.0000000000001875.

7 Fincham, G.W., Strauss, C., Montero-Marin, J. *et al.* (2023) 'Effect of breathwork on stress and mental health: A meta-analysis of randomised-controlled trials.' *Sci Rep 13*, 432. https://doi.org/10.1038/s41598-022-27247-y

8 Kennedy, D.O., Little, W. and Scholey, A.B. (2004) 'Attenuation of laboratory-induced stress in humans after acute administration of Melissa officinalis (lemon balm).' *Psychosomatic Medicine 66*, 4, 607–613. doi: 10.1097/01.psy.0000132877.72833.71.

9 Zanelati, T.V., Biojone, C., Moreira, F.A., Guimarães, F.S. and Joca, S.R. (2010) 'Antidepressant-like effects of cannabidiol in mice: Possible involvement of 5-HT1A receptors.' *British Journal of Pharmacology 159*, 1, 122–128. doi: 10.1111/j.1476-5381.2009.00521.x.

10 Zick, S.M., Wright, B.D., Sen, A. and Arndt, J.T. (2011) 'Preliminary examination of the efficacy and safety of a standardized chamomile extract for chronic primary insomnia: A randomized placebo-controlled pilot study.' *BMC Complementary and Alternative Medicine 11*, 78. doi: 10.1186/1472-6882-11-78.

Chapter 10

1 Erdélyi, A., Pálfi, E., Tűű, L.. *et al.* (2023) 'The Importance of Nutrition in Menopause and Perimenopause-A Review.' *Nutrients, 16*, 1, 27. doi: 10.3390/nu16010027.

2 Geraci, A., Calvani, R., Ferri, E., Marzetti, E., Arosio, B. and Cesari, M. (2021) 'Sarcopenia and menopause: The role of estradiol.' *Frontiers in Endocrinology 12*. https://doi.org/10.3389/fendo.2021.682012

3 Borack, M.S. and Volpi, E. (2016) 'Efficacy and safety of leucine supplementation in the elderly.' *The Journal of Nutrition 146*, 12, 2625S–2629S. doi: 10.3945/jn.116.230771.

4 Funderburk, L.K., Beretich, K.N., Chen, M.D. and Willoughby, D.S. (2020) 'Efficacy of L-leucine supplementation coupled with resistance training in untrained midlife women.' *Journal of the American College of Nutrition 39*, 4, 316–324. doi: 10.1080/07315724.2019.1650675.

5 Phillips, S.M. (2004) 'Protein requirements and supplementation in strength sports.' *Nutrition (Burbank, Los Angeles County, CA) 20*, 7–8, 689–695. doi: 10.1016/j.nut.2004.04.009.

6 Schoenfeld, B.J. and Aragon, A.A. (2018) 'How much protein can the body use in a single meal for muscle-building? Implications for daily protein distribution.' *Journal of the International Society of Sports Nutrition 15*, 10. doi: 10.1186/s12970-018-0215-1.

7 Jäger, R., Kerksick, C.M., Campbell, B.I., Cribb, P.J., *et al.* (2017) 'International Society of Sports Nutrition position stand: Protein and exercise.' *Journal of the International Society of Sports Nutrition 14*, 20. https://doi.org/10.1186/s12970-017-0177-8

8 Gameiro, C.M., Romão, F. and Castelo-Branco, C. (2010) 'Menopause and aging: Changes in the immune system – A review.' *Maturitas 67*, 4, 316–320. doi: 10.1016/j.maturitas.2010.08.003.

9 Ghosh, M., Rodriguez-Garcia, M. and Wira, C.R. (2014) 'The immune system in menopause: Pros and cons of hormone therapy.' *The Journal of Steroid Biochemistry and Molecular Biology 142*, 171–175. doi: 10.1016/j.jsbmb.2013.09.003.

10 Heitkemper, M.M. and Chang, L. (2009) 'Do fluctuations in ovarian hormones affect gastrointestinal symptoms in women with irritable bowel syndrome?' *Gender Medicine 6*, Suppl. 2, 152–167. doi: 10.1016/j.genm.2009.03.004.

11 Aziz, I., Hadjivassiliou, M. and Sanders, D.S. (2015) 'The spectrum of noncoeliac gluten sensitivity.' *Nature Reviews. Gastroenterology & Hepatology 12*, 9, 516–526. doi: 10.1038/nrgastro.2015.107.

12 Biesiekierski, J.R. and Iven, J. (2015) 'Non-coeliac gluten sensitivity: Piecing the puzzle together.' *United European Gastroenterology Journal 3*, 2, 160–165. doi: 10.1177/2050640615578388.

13 Pawlosky, R.J., Hibbeln, J.R., Novotny, J.A. and Salem Jr, N. (2001) 'Physiological compartmental analysis of α-linolenic acid metabolism in adult humans.' *Journal of Lipid Research 42*, 8, 1257–1265. PMID: 11483627.

14 Aguilera, C.M., Ramírez-Tortosa, M.C., Mesa, M.D. and Gil, A. (2001) 'Efectos protectores de los ácidos grasos monoinsaturados y poliinsaturados sobre el desarrollo de la enfermedad cardiovascular.' ['Protective effect of monounsaturated and polyunsaturated fatty acids on the development of cardiovascular disease.'] *Nutricion Hospitalaria* 16, 3, 78–91 [in Spanish]. PMID: 11475681

15 Hellhammer, J., Waladkhani, A.-R., Hero, T. and Buss, C. (2010) 'Effects of milk phospholipid on memory and psychological stress response.' *British Food Journal* 112, 10, 1124–1137. https://doi.org/10.1108/00070701011080258

16 Fischer, L.M., da Costa, K.A., Kwock, L., Galanko, J. and Zeisel, S.H. (2010) 'Dietary choline requirements of women: Effects of estrogen and genetic variation.' *The American Journal of Clinical Nutrition* 92, 5, 1113–1119. doi: 10.3945/ajcn.2010.30064.

17 Simopoulos, A.P. (2008) 'The importance of the omega-6/omega-3 fatty acid ratio in cardiovascular disease and other chronic diseases.' *Exp Biol Med (Maywood)* 233, 6, 674–688. doi: 10.3181/0711-MR-311.

18 Gill, S. and Panda, S. (2015) 'A smartphone app reveals erratic diurnal eating patterns in humans that can be modulated for health benefits.' *Cell Metabolism* 22, 5, 789–798. doi: 10.1016/j.cmet.2015.09.005.

19 Lin, S., Cienfuegos, S., Ezpeleta, M., Gabel, K., *et al.* (2023) 'Time-restricted eating without calorie counting for weight loss in a racially diverse population: A randomized controlled trial.' *Annals of Internal Medicine* 176, 7, 885–895. doi: 10.7326/M23-0052.

20 Gabel, K., Hoddy, K.K., Haggerty, N., Song, J., *et al.* (2018) 'Effects of 8-hour time restricted feeding on body weight and metabolic disease risk factors in obese adults: A pilot study.' *Nutrition and Healthy Aging 4*, 4, 345–353. doi: 10.3233/NHA-170036.

21 Milic, J., Glisic, M., Voortman, T., Borba, L.P., *et al.* (2018) 'Menopause, ageing, and alcohol use disorders in women.' *Maturitas* 111, 100–109. doi: 10.1016/j.maturitas.2018.03.006.

22 Daviet, R., Aydogan, G., Jagannathan, K., Spilka, N., *et al.* (2022) 'Associations between alcohol consumption and gray and white matter volumes in the UK Biobank.' *Nature Communications* 13, 1175. https://doi.org/10.1038/s41467-022-28735-5

23 Longnecker, M.P. and Tseng, M. (1998) 'Alcohol, hormones, and postmenopausal women.' *Alcohol Health and Research World* 22, 3, 185–189. PMID: 15706794.

Chapter 11

1 Zhao, H., Chen, J., Li, X., Sun, Q., Qin, P. and Wang, Q. (2019) 'Compositional and functional features of the female premenopausal and postmenopausal gut microbiota.' *FEBS Letters* 593, 2655–2664. doi: 10.1002/1873-3468.13527.

2 Peters, B.A., Lin, J., Qi, Q., *et al.* (2022) 'Menopause Is Associated with an Altered Gut Microbiome and Estrobolome, with Implications for Adverse Cardiometabolic Risk in the Hispanic Community Health Study/Study of Latinos.' *mSystems* 7, 3, e0027322. doi: 10.1128/msystems.00273-22.

3 Mayor, S. (2019) 'Eating more fibre linked to reduced risk of non-communicable diseases and death, review finds.' *BMJ 364*, l159. https://doi.org/10.1136/bmj.l159

4 McDonald, D., Hyde, E., Debelius, J.W., Morton, J.T., *et al.* (2018) 'American gut: An open platform for citizen science microbiome research.' *mSystems* 3, 3. doi: 10.1128/msystems.00031-18.

5 Kroenke, C.H., Caan, B.J., Stefanick, M.L., Anderson, G., *et al.* (2012) 'Effects of a dietary intervention and weight change on vasomotor symptoms in the Women's Health Initiative.' *Menopause (New York, N.Y.)* 19, 9, 980–988. doi: 10.1097/gme.0b013e31824f606e.

6 Özcan, H., Oskay, Ü. and Bodur, A.F. (2019) 'Effects of Kefir on Quality of Life and Sleep Disturbances in Postmenopausal Women.' *Holist Nurs Pract.* 33, 4, 207–213.

7 Kim, H.Y., Park, E.S., Choi, Y.S. *et al.* (2022) 'Kimchi improves irritable bowel syndrome: results of a randomized, double-blind placebo-controlled study.' *Food Nutr Res.*, 66. doi: 10.29219/fnr.v66.8268.

8 Cardona, F., Andrés-Lacueva, C., Tulipani, S., Tinahones, F.J. and Queipo-Ortuño, M.I. (2013) 'Benefits of polyphenols on gut microbiota and implications in human health.' *The Journal of Nutritional Biochemistry 24*, 8, 1415–1422. doi: 10.1016/j.jnutbio.2013.05.001.

9 Duda-Chodak, A. (2012) 'The inhibitory effect of polyphenols on human gut microbiota.' *Journal of Physiology and Pharmacology* 63, 5, 497–503. PMID: 23211303.

10 Filosa, S., Di Meo, F. and Crispi, S. (2018) 'Polyphenols-gut microbiota interplay and brain neuromodulation.' *Neural Regeneration Research 13*, 12, 2055–2059. doi: 10.4103/1673-5374.241429.

11 Reynolds, A., Mann J., Cummings, J., Winter, N., Mete, E. and Te Morenga, L. (2019) 'Carbohydrate quality and human health: A series of systematic reviews and me-

ta-analyses.' *The Lancet (London, England) 393*, 10170, 434–445. doi: 10.1016/S0140-6736(18)31809-9.

12 Bacciottini, L., Falchetti, A., Pampaloni, B., Bartolini, E., Carossino, A.M. and Brandi, M.L. (2007) 'Phytoestrogens: Food or drug?' *Clinical Cases in Mineral and Bone Metabolism 4*, 2, 123–130. PMID: 22461212.

13 Lissin, L.W. and Cooke, J.P. (2000) 'Phytoestrogens and cardiovascular health.' *Journal of the American College of Cardiology 35*, 6, 1403–1410. doi: 10.1016/s0735-1097(00)00590-8.

14 Desmawati, D. and Sulastri, D. (2019) 'Phytoestrogens and their health effect.' *Open Access Macedonian Journal of Medical Sciences 7*, 3, 495–499. doi: 10.3889/oamjms.2019.044.

15 Farhat, E.K., Sher, E.K., Džidić-Krivić, A., Banjari, I. and Sher, F. (2023) 'Functional biotransformation of phytoestrogens by gut microbiota with impact on cancer treatment.' *The Journal of Nutritional Biochemistry 118*, 109368. doi: 10.1016/j.jnutbio.2023.109368.

16 Messina, M. (2014) 'Soy foods, isoflavones, and the health of postmenopausal women.' *The American Journal of Clinical Nutrition 100*, Suppl. 1, 423S–30S. doi: 10.3945/ajcn.113.071464.

17 Calado, A., Neves, P.M., Santos, T. and Ravasco, P. (2018) 'The effect of flaxseed in breast cancer: A literature review.' *Frontiers in Nutrition 5*, 4. doi: 10.3389/fnut.2018.00004.

18 Adel-Mehraban, M.S., Tansaz, M., Mohammadi, M. and Yavari, M. (2022) 'Effects of pomegranate supplement on menopausal symptoms and quality of life in menopausal women: A double-blind randomized placebo-controlled trial.' *Complementary Therapies in Clinical Practice 46*, 101544. doi: 10.1016/j.ctcp.2022.101544.

Chapter 12

1 Feskens, E.J.M., Bailey, R., Bhutta, Z., Biesalski, H.K., *et al.* (2022) 'Women's health: Optimal nutrition throughout the lifecycle.' *European Journal of Nutrition 61*, Suppl. 1., 1–23. doi: 10.1007/s00394-022-02915-x.

2 Chester, R.C., Kling, J.M. and Manson, J.E. (2018) 'What the Women's Health Initiative has taught us about menopausal hormone therapy.' *Clinical Cardiology 41*, 2, 247–252. doi: 10.1002/clc.22891.

Subject Index

Sub-headings in *italics* indicate tables.

Author Index